MCQs in Clinical Pharmacy

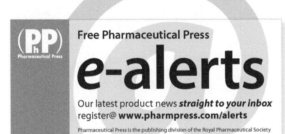

MCQs in Clinical Pharmacy

Edited by

Lilian M Azzopardi

BPharm (Hons), MPhil, PhD

Associate Professor
Department of Pharmacy
Faculty of Medicine and Surgery
University of Malta
Msida, Malta

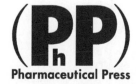

Pharmaceutical Press

Published by the Pharmaceutical Press

1 Lambeth High Street, London SE1 7JN, UK

© Pharmaceutical Press 2007

(**PP**) is a trade mark of Pharmaceutical Press
Pharmaceutical Press is the publishing division of the Royal Pharmaceutical
Society of Great Britain

First published 2007

Typeset by Type Study, Scarborough, North Yorkshire
Printed in Great Britain by TJ International, Padstow, Cornwall

ISBN 978 0 85369 666 7

A catalogue record for this book is available from the British Library.

Dedicated to the memory of Dr Cat and Mr Socrates, my departed cats, who kept persistent company during long hours of preparation of my publications

Contents

Foreword

The healthcare systems of most industrialised nations have a problem that needs the attention of pharmacists, if it is to be solved correctly. The problem is the poor quality of medicines use, and the solution includes increased pharmacist participation in medicines management.

Studies from many nations, conducted over many years, have shown the need for better management of drug therapy. This first became clear from 'process' studies showing some inappropriate prescribing, inadequate monitoring and advice, and patient non-adherence. Other studies took this a step further, and confirmed not only the prevalence of adverse outcomes of drug therapy, but also that such adverse outcomes often could have been prevented by more careful management. For example, the median preventability rate in one review was 59%.[1]

Mis-managed drug therapy may rank as one of the leading causes of hospital admission, because of adverse reactions, undertreatment, or non-treatment. The median rate of hospital admissions from preventable drug-related morbidity (PDRM)* in that review was 4.3%. This would rank PDRM with cancer, coronary heart disease, diabetes mellitus and asthma as a leading cause of hospital admissions in many countries. The rate of adverse outcomes among inpatients typically was 1.5%, and adverse drug events may prolong hospital stays by 2–4 days.[1,2]

* PDRM is much broader than adverse drug reactions (ADR) and somewhat broader than adverse drug events (ADE). Like ADE, PDRM includes errors and other problems in drug use as well as injury caused by the ineffective use or non-use of indicated drugs.

The possibilities of safer and more effective drug therapy have been clear, and evidence has been mounting about how to improve them. When pharmacists systematically cooperate with patients and other healthcare providers, with the objective of improving the outcomes of drug therapy, outcomes often improve and costs often decrease.[3,4]

The road to medicines management has not been like a broad, smooth motorway. Parts of it are, so to speak, unpaved and even unmarked. After nearly two decades of effort by practice researchers, practitioners and pharmaceutical societies throughout Europe and North America, some national programmes, for example, in the USA and the UK, have in effect recognised the need for pharmacists to participate fully in cooperative patient-centred systems. Success on the road ahead will require commitment, planning and effort.

How should pharmacists direct their efforts? Despite the conventional wisdom, prescribing problems are not the leading cause of preventable, drug-related hospital admissions. About 70% of such admissions involved some aspect of the management of ongoing drug therapy. Management of therapy included follow-up monitoring and detection of therapeutic problems, for example, treatment failures, laboratory tests not being done or not being acted upon, and moderate adverse drug reactions that were allowed to become so severe that they necessitated admission. Problems with prescribing, including drug choice, dosage and route accounted for about 16%; drug distribution and administration, including patient non-adherence, accounted for about 13%. Among inpatients, the situation was roughly the opposite: most problems involved prescribing and the fewest involved follow up.[2]

As prescribing is not a leading cause of PDRM in ambulatory care, simple prescribing improvement programmes such as formularies are ineffective when the goal is to improve patient outcomes or reduce total costs or care. Likewise, compliance improvement programmes may improve medication-taking behaviour but rarely show a positive effect on outcomes. The outcomes of drug therapy in ambulatory care can be improved by increasing organised (systematic) cooperation among pharmacists, physicians and patients. Such changes are associated with improved outcomes and reduced total costs of care in many studies.[3,4] Even modest improvements in customary arrangements may be associated with improved outcomes, lower total costs of care, or both.

Pharmacists are strategically important, but they are not essential. If pharmacy is not up to the task, others will surely step forward. Our public image is favourable, but has been somewhat dated. Patients and policymakers in some countries have now begun to change their impression of pharmacists, from a dispenser to a drug expert who can help patients make the best use of their medicines.

Pharmaceutical education, and in some cases, re-education in pharmacotherapeutics will be one essential ingredient in pharmacy's efforts. Some pharmacists, however, do not intervene, even when they see and understand a drug therapy problem, its causes and its solutions. I have long suspected that one underlying cause of such inaction is a lack of confidence, as if pharmacists do not appreciate their own knowledge and how much they can contribute to patient welfare. If this book helps pharmacists to focus, recognise and appreciate their clinical knowledge, it will be a useful addition to that enterprise.

The road to pharmaceutical care and medicines management may be uncharted, but it does not go through a minefield where we can lose everything from one error. We are not in a game that we can lose if our failures outnumber our successes. We are like the pilot in the first chapter of Tom Wolfe's *The Right Stuff*. We need to keep trying until we find what succeeds, and then take the next step. We are succeeding.

Charles D Hepler, PhD
Distinguished Professor Emeritus
College of Pharmacy
The University of Florida
Gainesville, Florida, USA
February 2007

References

1   Winterstein A, Sauer B C, Hepler C D *et al*. Preventable drug-related hospital admissions and morbidity in hospitalized patients – a meta-analysis of prevalence reports. *Ann Pharmacother* 2002; 36: 1238–1248.

2   Hepler C D, Segal R. Chapters 2–3 in *Preventing Medication Errors and Improving Drug Therapy Outcomes through System Management*. Boca Raton, Florida: CRC Press, 2003.

3   Hepler C D, Segal R. Chapter 9 in *Preventing Medication Errors and Improving Drug Therapy Outcomes through System Management*. Boca Raton, Florida: CRC Press, 2003.

4   MacKinnon N J. How much evidence is enough? *Can Pharm J* 2002; (July–Aug): 25–29.

Preface

This book edited by Lilian Azzopardi is aimed at helping pharmacy students and pharmacists to grasp the principles of clinical pharmacy during their career development. The book presents 320 multiple-choice questions, and for each question a concise answer is given. It is highly practical, short and to the point. As a seasoned examiner, I would recommend it as a useful revision aid.

Another characteristic of the book is that it shifts the focus from theory to clinical applications, reflecting the growing trend to change critical appraisals into clinical action. The examples feature real case histories, providing the opportunity to simulate actual practice, where multiple problems are presented, decisions need to be taken, and the required monitoring of the patient may be influenced by the occurrence of concurrent disease states.

This context, where multiple problem scenarios are presented, stimulates the candidate to think and generate ideas similar to those required in practice, where an holistic approach is required for optimum management. The questions addressing the cases are developed so as to stress the general principles and concepts that can be applied to other situations, as well as to discuss issues that are particular to the patient.

The uniqueness of this publication lies in the fact that the authors were able to produce a book which presents problems that are taken from contemporary clinical practice. It induces candidates to acquire those skills that are needed to tackle clinical pharmacy practice issues effectively.

I am confident that the book reflects the enthusiasm Lilian and her colleagues have for the practice of clinical pharmacy and for developing problem-based learning approaches in teaching and career development. Clinical pharmacy is the basis for pharmaceutical care. Therefore it is very relevant that the book extends its parameters to include practical issues related to the development of pharmaceutical care plans, drug therapy selection and drug therapy monitoring. Again, as it draws strongly on the practical aspect, the book should also be used by pharmacists for continuing professional development in the area of clinical pharmacy, including those serving society in all aspects of pharmaceutical care.

Professor Godfrey LaFerla
Dean, Faculty of Medicine and Surgery
Head, Department of Surgery
University of Malta
Malta
February 2007

Acknowledgements

In the development of the concept of this publication, I have drawn on my experience in teaching and practicing clinical pharmacy. Looking back, I can state that I have been able to develop these skills by working in collaboration with a number of colleagues, mostly from the Faculty of Medicine and Surgery at the University of Malta. Most importantly I am indebted to Professor Anthony Serracino-Inglott and to Dr Maurice Zarb-Adami from the Department of Pharmacy, who have inspired me through their dedication for pharmacy to develop clinical pharmacy skills that put the patient in focus and to perform effective teaching of students. They had vision about my enthusiasm for providing useful student revision aids.

Together with Professor Steve Hudson, University of Strathclyde and Professor Sam Salek, University of Cardiff, I have discussed at length clinical pharmacy practice in different scenarios. This book reflects the philosophies of my colleagues Anthony Serracino-Inglott, Maurice Zarb-Adami, Steve Hudson and Sam Salek. Indeed it was again a pleasure for all of us to work together for a third publication.

I am especially indebted to Professor Roger Ellul-Micallef, Head of the Department of Clinical Pharmacology and Therapeutics at the University of Malta for his very relevant comments on the material presented in the book. Special thanks go to Dr Bernard Coleiro, Senior Registrar, Department of Medicine at St Luke's Hospital, to my sister Louise Azzopardi, clinical pharmacist at St Luke's Hospital and to Dr Mark Grech, Medical Officer, St Luke's Hospital for reviewing the text.

My appreciation goes to Professor Godfrey LaFerla, Dean of the Faculty of Medicine and Surgery at the University of Malta and to Professor Charles Hepler, Emeritus Professor at the University of Florida who dedicated time from their very demanding schedule to contribute the preface and the foreword of the book. In addition I would like to thank Professor Juanito Camilleri, Rector of the University of Malta for his support.

Thanks go to colleagues and staff at the Faculty of Medicine and Surgery and to pharmacy students for their enthusiasm towards clinical pharmacy.

Completion of a book is not possible without the support of the publisher. I would like to thank the team from Pharmaceutical Press led by Christina DeBono and Louise McIndoe for their input and for keeping up with my exacting demands.

Finally thanks go to my family for their support.

About the editor

Lilian M. Azzopardi studied pharmacy at the University of Malta, Faculty of Medicine and Surgery. In 1994 she took up a position at the Department of Pharmacy, University of Malta as a teaching and research assistant. Professor Azzopardi completed an MPhil on the development of formulary systems for community pharmacy in 1995, and in 1999 she graduated a PhD. Her PhD thesis led to the publication of the book *Validation Instruments for Community Pharmacy: pharmaceutical care for the third millennium* published in 2000 by Pharmaceutical Products Press, USA. She worked together with Professor Anthony Serracino-Inglott, who was a pioneer in the introduction of clinical pharmacy in the late sixties. In 2003 Dr Azzopardi edited the book *MCQs in Pharmacy Practice* published by the Pharmaceutical Press, UK which was followed in 2006 by the book *Further MCQs in Pharmacy Practice*.

Lilian Azzopardi is currently an associate professor in pharmacy practice at the Department of Pharmacy, University of Malta and is responsible for coordinating several aspects of the teaching of pharmacy practice, including clinical pharmacy for undergraduate and postgraduate students, as well as supervising a number of pharmacy projects and dissertations in the field. She is an examiner at the University of Malta for students following the pharmacy course and is an assessor in determining suitability to practice.

Lilian Azzopardi was, for a short period, interim director of the European Society of Clinical Pharmacy (ESCP) and is currently coordinator of the ESCP newsletter. She served as a member of the

Working Group on Quality Care Standards within the Community Pharmacy Section of the International Pharmaceutical Federation (FIP). She was a member of the Pharmacy Board, the licensing authority for pharmacy in Malta for a number of years and Registrar of the Malta College of Pharmacy Practice, which is responsible for continuing education. In 1997 she was given an award by the FIP Foundation for Education and Research, and in 1999 received the ESCP German Research and Education Foundation grant. She has practised clinical pharmacy in the hospital setting and she practises in community pharmacy.

Lilian Azzopardi has published several papers on clinical pharmacy and pharmaceutical care, and has actively participated at congresses organised by FIP, ESCP, the Royal Pharmaceutical Society of Great Britain, the American Pharmaceutical Association and the American Society of Health-System Pharmacists. She has been invited to give lectures and short courses in this area in several universities. In particular she is course organiser and tutor on the Patient Centred Clinical Pharmacy course arranged annually by ESCP in Malta since 2001, under the leadership of Professor Steve Hudson, in which over 100 clinical pharmacy teachers and practitioners from different countries have taken part.

Contributors

Lilian M Azzopardi BPharm (Hons.), MPhil, PhD
Associate Professor, Department of Pharmacy, Faculty of Medicine and Surgery, University of Malta, Msida, Malta

Stephen A Hudson MPharm, FRPharmS
Professor of Pharmaceutical Care, Division of Pharmaceutical Sciences, Strathclyde Institute of Pharmacy and Biomedical Sciences, University of Strathclyde, Glasgow, UK

Sam Salek PhD, RPh, MFPM (Hon)
Professor and Director, Centre for Socioeconomic Research, Welsh School of Pharmacy, Cardiff, UK

Anthony Serracino-Inglott BPharm, PharmD
Professor and Head of Department, Department of Pharmacy, University of Malta, Msida, Malta

Maurice Zarb-Adami BPharm, PhD
Senior Lecturer, Department of Pharmacy, University of Malta, Msida, Malta

Introduction

In the years following the Second World War, the contribution that pharmacists could make to the successful treatment of patients, by being involved in the selection of that treatment, began to be appreciated.

The subject of clinical pharmacy was developed in the late 1960s to help pharmacists meet the challenge of acquiring an education that places the patient at the centre of their professional activity. This book should help to enhance the clinical aspects of pharmacy education.

In today's climate of burgeoning information and complex clinical issues, a career in clinical pharmacy is more demanding than ever. Increasingly, training in clinical aspects of pharmacy must prepare pharmacists to seek and synthesise the necessary information and to apply that information successfully. The questions in this book are designed not only to provide examples that may be asked in clinical pharmacy examinations, but also to provide a logical framework for organising, learning, reviewing and applying the conceptual and factual information to the clinical scenario.

The clinical pharmacist must be able to select the relevant information and apply it effectively to the clinical situation. The experienced clinical pharmacist has acquired some clinical perspective through practice: we hope that this book (especially the case studies) imparts some of this to the relatively inexperienced. The format and contents are designed for the examination candidate but the same approach to problems should help the practising clinical pharmacist in the lifelong education required in everyday work.

The book is not meant to be used as an introduction to clinical pharmacy for the undergraduate, because the questions assume much basic knowledge, and considerable detailed information had to be omitted from the answers. Although the book has a number of appendices giving definitions of conditions and terminology, abbreviations and acronyms, and clinical laboratory data, these are intended to serve as an aide-memoire; they are not meant to replace the need for continually consulting references in the field.

The questions presented in the four tests are divided into two parts: essential background information, which is covered in approximately the first 25% of the questions in each test; and the clinical approach, as seen in the case studies. In the case studies we have considered the situation that a candidate meets in a clinical scenario. Although the cases are all specific, by finishing the four tests the candidate should have learnt that the best way to carry out these exercises is to follow a systematic approach.

Most of the cases dealt with in these tests involve circumstances met with in daily practice, such as pulmonary oedema, heart failure, hypothyroidism, dehydration and diabetes. A large number of common diseases are included but certainly not all. We highly recommend reading the short explanations of the answers, even when a correct answer is achieved, as we emphasise points that are understressed in some textbooks.

We have also included a couple of cases that are relatively not so common in everyday practice. It is necessary for the clinical pharmacist to know about these and to be capable of reaching a solution to the presented problem. It is to be remembered that in some scenarios clinical pharmacist services are available on an as-and-when-required basis. In such a case, the clinical pharmacist is often consulted when a rare case is met with, especially by junior doctors. An example from this book is the case describing an overdose of promethazine and alcohol withdrawal symptoms.

Supplementary reading is essential to understand the basic pathology involved in these cases, but the information given in the short answers is probably all that needs to be known by the candidate, and should be sufficient to provide the knowledge required to reach the correct answer. It should be noted that an awareness of some rare situations is essential, because it is often in such cases that the availability of a clinical pharmacist could lead to the correct treatment; it may be instrumental in improving the prognosis and on occasions may even be life saving.

Questions on such conditions are also important for candidates preparing for examinations, because examiners tend to include a rare case or two, to avoid setting a stereotyped examination involving the same diseases.

We have not attempted to cover all aspects of clinical pharmacy but – by cross-referencing between one case and another, and by using the questions that do not involve case studies – only a few subjects were omitted. This is reinforced by a cursory look at the indices, on generic names, subject and conditions, in addition to the cases index. Highly specialized situations, such as those occurring in oncology, were thought to be unsuitable for inclusion here. Psychiatry and dermatology are two areas that are often forgotten by clinical pharmacy students during revision; both subjects are very relevant to pharmacy.

Clinical pharmacists need to understand basic facts on diseases and the relevance of laboratory tests (including common abbreviations and acronyms), to be able to contribute their expertise on therapeutic management in the clinical scenario. The first questions in each test cover these requirements, which are needed to tackle the comprehensive case study questions.

Before tackling the case studies questions, it is worth ensuring that you can answer correctly the questions in the beginning of the test. Knowledge of the meaning of medical terms such as hypoxia, tachypnoea, myopathy and dysphasia, the significance of laboratory tests such as INR, HbA1c, BUN, TSH, LFT and MCV and of the meaning of abbreviations such as PMH, O/E, PC and FH is also tested in the questions. It may be wise to read through appendices A, B and C, which give the meaning of medical terms, abbreviations and the significance of laboratory tests, before attempting the questions.

Other short questions require a knowledge of side-effects of medicines, disease symptoms and reasons for the occurrence of certain reactions, such as resistance to drug therapy. The specific advice that needs to be given to patients in relation to the use of particular medicines, such as when dispensing isosorbide dinitrate, is emphasised throughout the text. Clinical pharmacists ought to have a thorough, detailed knowledge of drugs, including indications, contraindications, monitoring requirements, dosage regimens, adverse effects and when reporting is required, and of different classifications, such as chemical or therapeutic. A list of all drugs mentioned in the text is conveniently presented in the generic name index. You can use this index as a self-test to confirm your preparedness by answering these questions: (1) when is this drug indicated?; (2) what are the contraindications or cautions?; (3) what adverse effects may occur and which of these require early or immediate attention?; (4) how is the drug classified and what is its mechanism of action?; (5) does the drug have particular properties that are of great relevance, such as tolerance, addiction, teratogenicity and the possibility of resistance developing?

In this book our aim is to base questions on those aspects of clinical pharmacy that bear most relevance to practice and which enjoy wide general acceptance. It is hoped that the questions will be useful not only to candidates preparing for examinations, both undergraduate and postgraduate, but also to practitioners as a means of continuing education. We have tried to avoid excessive detail in the way of figures, laboratory investigations and in the facts given; in general those that are included are of value and essential to tackle the question.

The purpose of this book is to revise aspects of clinical pharmacy, to prepare for examinations and to apply pharmacy concepts in continued self-education at undergraduate and postgraduate level. It has been our experience that students who understand the basic pharmaceutical sciences such as physiology, biochemistry, medicinal chemistry, pharmaceutics and pharmacology have little difficulty in practising as clinical pharmacists, whereas those who have learned their basic subjects in a parrot-like fashion are unlikely to thrive in clinical pharmacy, as making good use of the basic sciences is a requirement. This book therefore also serves to show how essential the basic sciences are to perform well in clinical pharmacy.

An advantage of having an MCQs book as a revision tool is that during a revision exercise you must commit yourself to an opinion – using MCQs you have the opportunity to confirm that the opinion is correct. When mistaken, with the aid of the Answers section, you can pursue the matter until you understand why your answer was incorrect. The Answers section should also serve to reinforce the correct impressions. We do not profess that clinical pharmacy could be reduced to a mere collection of question and answer statements, which are all 100% true or false. However we hope that you will find, on investigation and reflection, that most of the statements correlate to real-case scenarios, where a decision often must be taken in the manner reflected in the text.

Revision checklist

For each test, write the number of the question and your answer on a separate sheet of paper, then after going through all the questions in the test, compare your answers with those in the book.

Refer to Appendix D for feedback on those questions that you did not answer correctly, to be able to compare your ability with a cohort of students.

Appendix A includes definitions of medical terms included in the book, while Appendix B lists abbreviations and acronyms. Appendix C presents laboratory test results for parameters that are mentioned in the book.

Checklist

This checklist should help students identify areas that need to be covered when preparing for an exam in clinical pharmacy.

- *Patient assessment:* physical assessment skills, laboratory and diagnostic information
- *Therapeutic planning:* problem identification, pharmaceutical care plan, selection of therapeutic regimens, patient monitoring
- *Monitoring drug therapy:* patient counselling, adverse effects, baseline tests
- *Drug information:* patient counselling, cautionary labels, cautions, contraindications
- *Responding to symptoms:* presentation of conditions, diagnosis, referrals, use of non-prescription medicines, patient counselling

Test 1

Questions

Questions 1-6

Directions: Each group of questions below consists of five lettered headings followed by a list of numbered questions. For each numbered question select the one heading that is most closely related to it. Each heading may be used once, more than once, or not at all.

Questions 1-3 concern the following:

A ☐ MCHC
B ☐ lymphocytes
C ☐ HbA1c
D ☐ INR
E ☐ thrombocytes

Select, from A to E, which one of the above:

Q1 may be decreased in iron deficiency anaemia

Q2 may have an increased value in viral infections

Q3 may have a decreased value in idiopathic thrombocytopenia purpura

Questions 4–6 concern the following:

A ☐ tachypnoea
B ☐ hypoxia
C ☐ afterload
D ☐ myopathy
E ☐ dysphasia

Select, from A to E, which one of the above is manifested by:

Q4 muscle weakness and muscle wasting

Q5 rapid rate of breathing

Q6 an impairment of the language aspect of speech

Questions 7–26

Directions: For each of the questions below, ONE or MORE of the responses is (are) correct. Decide which of the responses is (are) correct. Then choose:

A ☐ if 1, 2 and 3 are correct
B ☐ if 1 and 2 only are correct
C ☐ if 2 and 3 only are correct
D ☐ if 1 only is correct
E ☐ if 3 only is correct

Directions summarised				
A	**B**	**C**	**D**	**E**
1, 2, 3	1, 2 only	2, 3 only	1 only	3 only

Q7   Drugs that may cause plasma sodium electrolyte disturbances include:

1   ❑ prednisolone
2   ❑ salbutamol
3   ❑ propranolol

Q8   Conditions that may give rise to muscular or joint pain include:

1   ❑ Paget's disease
2   ❑ neuropathy
3   ❑ haemophilia

Q9   Symptoms that may indicate neoplastic disease if unexplained include:

1   ❑ skin ulceration
2   ❑ unexplained fractures
3   ❑ general debility

Q10   Possible causes of resistance to cytotoxic chemotherapy include:

1   ❑ increased cellular uptake
2   ❑ increased repair of DNA damage
3   ❑ poor penetration into tumour

Q11   In Parkinson's disease the patient could be referred for services from the:

1   ❑ speech therapy department
2   ❑ physiotherapy department
3   ❑ pain management team

Q12   Ultrasound scanning:

1   ❑ is associated with no radiation dose
2   ❑ may be used to define organ size and shape
3   ❑ can detect arterial blood flow to the organ

Q13   Creatinine clearance:

1   ☐ is an index used to measure glomerular filtration rate
2   ☐ measurement involves a 24-hour urine collection
3   ☐ measurement requires 24-hour monitoring of plasma creatinine

Q14   Patients receiving isosorbide dinitrate should be advised that:

1   ☐ occurrence of headaches tends to decrease with continued therapy
2   ☐ tablets should be discarded 8 weeks after opening the container
3   ☐ tablets should be stored in glass containers

Q15   Adrenaline:

1   ☐ is used in cardiac arrest
2   ☐ administration requires monitoring of blood pressure
3   ☐ results in a fall in blood pressure

Q16   Methadone:

1   ☐ requires multiple dosing in a day
2   ☐ is addictive
3   ☐ is an opioid agonist

Q17   Patients receiving tamoxifen should be advised:

1   ☐ that hot flushes may occur
2   ☐ that menstrual irregularities may occur
3   ☐ to report sudden breathlessness and any pain in the calf

Q18   Parenteral sodium bicarbonate:

1   ☐ raises blood pH
2   ☐ is indicated in metabolic acidosis
3   ☐ may be used in hypomagnesaemia

Q19   Phytomenadione:

1   ☐   is a lipid-soluble analogue of vitamin K
2   ☐   promotes hepatic synthesis of active prothrombin
3   ☐   is indicated in babies at birth to prevent vitamin K deficiency bleeding

Q20   Enoxaparin:

1   ☐   cannot be used at the same dose as heparin
2   ☐   thrombocytopenia may occur with its use
3   ☐   agents that affect haemostasis should be used with care

Q21   Patients receiving oral isotretinoin should be advised:

1   ☐   to avoid pregnancy
2   ☐   to avoid wax epilation during treatment
3   ☐   to use a lip balm regularly

Q22   A patient who will be undergoing a colonoscopy is advised to:

1   ☐   use a topical haemorrhoid preparation before admission
2   ☐   take a bowel cleansing preparation
3   ☐   avoid solid food on previous day

Q23   In which of the following cases is referral recommended:

1   ☐   a paediatric patient with a history of asthma who presents with a chest infection
2   ☐   a patient receiving diuretics who presents with symptoms of a heat stroke
3   ☐   a tourist who presents with acute diarrhoea

Q24 Anti-infectives that are used in the triple-therapy regimens to eradicate *Helicobacter pylori* include:

1 ☐ metronidazole
2 ☐ clarithromycin
3 ☐ telithromycin

Q25 In HIV infection:

1 ☐ accumulation of mutations associated with drug resistance may occur
2 ☐ drug resistance testing is not possible
3 ☐ monotherapy is preferred

Q26 Diabetic ketoacidosis:

1 ☐ is associated with insulin deficiency
2 ☐ may be precipitated by a severe infection
3 ☐ causes retinopathy

Questions 27–80

Directions: These questions involve cases. Read the case description or patient profile and answer the questions. For questions with one or more correct answers, follow the key given with each question. For the other questions, only one answer is correct – give the corresponding answer.

Questions 27–31 involve the following case:

PS is hospitalised with pulmonary oedema. Patient is started on metolazone 2.5 mg daily and bumetanide 2 mg bd iv

Q27   Signs and symptoms of pulmonary oedema include:

1   ❑   weight loss
2   ❑   dyspnoea
3   ❑   cough

A   ❑   1, 2, 3
B   ❑   1, 2 only
C   ❑   2, 3 only
D   ❑   1 only
E   ❑   3 only

Q28   Precipitants of acute pulmonary oedema include:

1   ❑   hypothyroidism
2   ❑   excessive infusion rate
3   ❑   heart failure

A   ❑   1, 2, 3
B   ❑   1, 2 only
C   ❑   2, 3 only
D   ❑   1 only
E   ❑   3 only

Q29   Parameters that are monitored during metolazone therapy include:

1   ❑   body weight
2   ❑   electrolytes
3   ❑   LFTs

A   ❑   1, 2, 3
B   ❑   1, 2 only
C   ❑   2, 3 only
D   ❑   1 only
E   ❑   3 only

Q30   Metolazone and bumetanide:

  A   ☐ reduce the blood volume
  B   ☐ produce a euphoric state
  C   ☐ cause sedation
  D   ☐ control bronchospasm
  E   ☐ prevent embolisation

Q31   When PS is stabilised, the therapeutic plan should consider:

  1   ☐ stopping metolazone treatment
  2   ☐ changing bumetanide to an oral formulation
  3   ☐ starting co-amoxiclav

  A   ☐ 1, 2, 3
  B   ☐ 1, 2 only
  C   ☐ 2, 3 only
  D   ☐ 1 only
  E   ☐ 3 only

Questions 32–38 involve the following case:

CA is a 77-year-old patient who is admitted to hospital with infected multiple sores and who is complaining of polyuria and weakness. CA presented with reduced skin turgor, dehydration, tremor and in a confused state. CA has a past medical history of diabetes. Her general practitioner has started her the day before on ciprofloxacin 250 mg bd and fusidic acid cream bd. Diabetes was managed through dietary control and CA was not taking antidiabetic drugs. On admission, CA is started on:

  glibenclamide 2.5 mg daily
  ciprofloxacin 500 mg bd
  sodium chloride 0.9% iv infusion
  haloperidol 0.5 mg bd

On admission: random blood glucose level 12 mmol/l
  blood pressure 125/78 mmHg

Q32 Management aims for CA include:

1 ☐ rehydration
2 ☐ control of hyperglycaemia
3 ☐ management of hypertension

A ☐ 1, 2, 3
B ☐ 1, 2 only
C ☐ 2, 3 only
D ☐ 1 only
E ☐ 3 only

Q33 Parameters that need to be monitored to assess outcomes of therapy include:

1 ☐ urine output
2 ☐ blood glucose monitoring
3 ☐ thyroid function tests

A ☐ 1, 2, 3
B ☐ 1, 2 only
C ☐ 2, 3 only
D ☐ 1 only
E ☐ 3 only

Q34 Signs which indicate that the diabetes in CA is uncontrolled include:

1 ☐ infected sores
2 ☐ reduced skin turgor
3 ☐ tremor

A ☐ 1, 2, 3
B ☐ 1, 2 only
C ☐ 2, 3 only
D ☐ 1 only
E ☐ 3 only

Q35   Pharmacist intervention with regards to therapy started on admission includes:

1 ☐ increase dose of ciprofloxacin
2 ☐ review sodium chloride infusion
3 ☐ rationale for haloperidol treatment

A ☐ 1, 2, 3
B ☐ 1, 2 only
C ☐ 2, 3 only
D ☐ 1 only
E ☐ 3 only

Q36   As regards glibenclamide therapy:

A ☐ gliclazide is preferred in this patient
B ☐ the dose could be increased to 10 mg daily
C ☐ the drug is administered in the afternoon
D ☐ the drug reduces insulin secretion
E ☐ it restores beta-cell activity

Q37   When the patient is discharged, advice includes:

1 ☐ consuming small, frequent regular meals
2 ☐ taking glibenclamide regularly
3 ☐ using fusidic acid cream daily

A ☐ 1, 2, 3
B ☐ 1, 2 only
C ☐ 2, 3 only
D ☐ 1 only
E ☐ 3 only

Q38   Onset of hypoglycaemia in CA could be precipitated by:

1   ❑ missed doses of glibenclamide
2   ❑ excess dietary intake
3   ❑ skipped meals

A   ❑ 1, 2, 3
B   ❑ 1, 2 only
C   ❑ 2, 3 only
D   ❑ 1 only
E   ❑ 3 only

Questions 39–41 involve the following case:

BD is a 34-year-old patient admitted with an overdose of promethazine and alcohol withdrawal symptoms. Patient has a history of alcohol abuse.

Q39   Symptoms that could occur due to promethazine overdose include:

1   ❑ drowsiness
2   ❑ headache
3   ❑ blurred vision

A   ❑ 1, 2, 3
B   ❑ 1, 2 only
C   ❑ 2, 3 only
D   ❑ 1 only
E   ❑ 3 only

Q40   Promethazine is an:

A   ☐ antidepressant
B   ☐ antipsychotic
C   ☐ antihistamine
D   ☐ analgesic
E   ☐ anxiolytic

Q41   A drug that can be used in alcohol withdrawal is:

A   ☐ beclometasone
B   ☐ chlorphenamine
C   ☐ lithium
D   ☐ diazepam
E   ☐ risperidone

Questions 42–44 involve the following case:

MB is a 58-year-old woman who presents with a prescription for simvastatin
10 mg daily. Her current medication is atenolol 50 mg daily. MB suffered a heart
attack last year.

Q42   MB is advised:

1   ☐ to report any muscle pain or weakness
2   ☐ to take simvastatin at night
3   ☐ to stop taking atenolol

A   ☐ 1, 2, 3
B   ☐ 1, 2 only
C   ☐ 2, 3 only
D   ☐ 1 only
E   ☐ 3 only

Q43   Side-effects to be expected with simvastatin include:

1   ☐ headache
2   ☐ nausea
3   ☐ abdominal pain

A   ☐ 1, 2, 3
B   ☐ 1, 2 only
C   ☐ 2, 3 only
D   ☐ 1 only
E   ☐ 3 only

Q44   Recommendations made to MB include:

1   ☐ follow moderate exercise
2   ☐ adopt a low-fat diet
3   ☐ take atenolol 2 h before simvastatin

A   ☐ 1, 2, 3
B   ☐ 1, 2 only
C   ☐ 2, 3 only
D   ☐ 1 only
E   ☐ 3 only

Questions 45–47 involve the following case:

GD is a 72-year-old female whose current medication is:
    aspirin 75 mg daily
    dipyridamole 100 mg tds
    timotol 0.5% both eyes 2 drops bd
    lactulose 20 ml daily

Q45   Dipyridamole:

1   ❑ cannot be used in combination with low-dose aspirin
2   ❑ is used for prophylaxis of thromboembolism
3   ❑ may cause increased bleeding during or after surgery

A   ❑ 1, 2, 3
B   ❑ 1, 2 only
C   ❑ 2, 3 only
D   ❑ 1 only
E   ❑ 3 only

Q46   Lactulose:

1   ❑ dose needs to be reviewed as the maximum adult daily dose is 5 ml
2   ❑ should not be used for more than 5 days
3   ❑ is used to maintain bowel evacuation

A   ❑ 1, 2, 3
B   ❑ 1, 2 only
C   ❑ 2, 3 only
D   ❑ 1 only
E   ❑ 3 only

Q47   GD is receiving medications for:

1   ❑ glaucoma
2   ❑ diarrhoea
3   ❑ osteoporosis

A   ❑ 1, 2, 3
B   ❑ 1, 2 only
C   ❑ 2, 3 only
D   ❑ 1 only
E   ❑ 3 only

Questions 48–53 involve the following case:

SP is a 64-year-old patient who is admitted to hospital with tiredness, shortness of breath and ankle oedema. She has a medical history of congestive heart failure. SP was intolerant to enalapril owing to the development of a cough. Her medications on admission are:

spironolactone 12.5 mg daily

losartan 25 mg daily

Q48   The therapeutic aims for SP are:

1   ❑   to control symptoms of heart failure
2   ❑   to control oedema
3   ❑   to control diabetes

A   ❑   1, 2, 3
B   ❑   1, 2 only
C   ❑   2, 3 only
D   ❑   1 only
E   ❑   3 only

Q49   Spironolactone:

1   ❑   reduces symptoms and mortality
2   ❑   dose may be increased to 25 mg daily
3   ❑   is an aldosterone antagonist

A   ❑   1, 2, 3
B   ❑   1, 2 only
C   ❑   2, 3 only
D   ❑   1 only
E   ❑   3 only

Q50   Monitoring required because of spironolactone treatment involves:

1   ❑ serum creatinine
2   ❑ serum potassium
3   ❑ thyroid function

A   ❑ 1, 2, 3
B   ❑ 1, 2 only
C   ❑ 2, 3 only
D   ❑ 1 only
E   ❑ 3 only

Q51   Losartan:

1   ❑ is an angiotensin-II receptor antagonist
2   ❑ exhibits a lower incidence of cough as a side-effect
      compared with enalapril
3   ❑ dose may be increased to 50 mg daily

A   ❑ 1, 2, 3
B   ❑ 1, 2 only
C   ❑ 2, 3 only
D   ❑ 1 only
E   ❑ 3 only

Q52   Digoxin is used in patients with heart failure:

1   ❑ because it decreases myocardial intracellular ionic calcium
2   ❑ when there is atrial fibrillation
3   ❑ because it exerts a positive inotropic effect

A   ❑ 1, 2, 3
B   ❑ 1, 2 only
C   ❑ 2, 3 only
D   ❑ 1 only
E   ❑ 3 only

Q53   Parameters to be monitored when digoxin therapy is started:

1   ❑   plasma digoxin concentration
2   ❑   plasma potassium measurement
3   ❑   plasma sodium measurement

A   ❑   1, 2, 3
B   ❑   1, 2 only
C   ❑   2, 3 only
D   ❑   1 only
E   ❑   3 only

Questions 54–57 involve the following case:

LB is a 55-year-old male patient who developed vesicles unilaterally around his waist. LB complained of a stabbing irritation in the area. LB is prescribed aciclovir 800 mg five times daily for 5 days.

Q54   The likely diagnosis for LB is:

A   ❑   prickly heat
B   ❑   herpes zoster infection
C   ❑   herpes labialis infection
D   ❑   cytomegalovirus infection
E   ❑   hepatitis B infection

Q55   Patient should be advised:

1   ❑   to take doses at regular intervals
2   ❑   to avoid exposure to sunlight
3   ❑   to wash hands thoroughly after drug administration

A ☐ 1, 2, 3
B ☐ 1, 2 only
C ☐ 2, 3 only
D ☐ 1 only
E ☐ 3 only

Q56 Side-effects that may be expected include:

1 ☐ headache
2 ☐ nausea
3 ☐ diarrhoea

A ☐ 1, 2, 3
B ☐ 1, 2 only
C ☐ 2, 3 only
D ☐ 1 only
E ☐ 3 only

Q57 Adjuvant therapy that may be used for LB include(s):

1 ☐ calamine lotion
2 ☐ amitriptyline
3 ☐ ergotamine

A ☐ 1, 2, 3
B ☐ 1, 2 only
C ☐ 2, 3 only
D ☐ 1 only
E ☐ 3 only

Questions 58–63 involve the following case:

AD is a 39-year-old female with bacterial endocarditis. She is started on gentamicin 80 mg iv twice daily and penicillin G iv 1.8 g every 6 h.

Q58   Penicillin G is:

A   ☐   phenoxymethylpenicillin
B   ☐   benzylpenicillin
C   ☐   penicillin V
D   ☐   piperacillin
E   ☐   pivmecillinam

Q59   Penicillin G is available in 600 mg vials. How many vials are required for each dose?

A   ☐   0.5
B   ☐   1
C   ☐   2
D   ☐   3
E   ☐   30

Q60   Penicillin G:

1   ☐   is bacteriostatic
2   ☐   is bactericidal
3   ☐   can be given as an intramuscular injection

A   ☐   1, 2, 3
B   ☐   1, 2 only
C   ☐   2, 3 only
D   ☐   1 only
E   ☐   3 only

Q61 Gentamicin:

1 ☐ has a broad spectrum of activity
2 ☐ is contraindicated in hepatic impairment
3 ☐ therapy may be changed to oral administration when the patient is stabilised

A ☐ 1, 2, 3
B ☐ 1, 2 only
C ☐ 2, 3 only
D ☐ 1 only
E ☐ 3 only

Patient developed a rash and started complaining of generalised itch after the administration of the drugs.

Q62 A possible reason for these symptoms is:

1 ☐ allergy to gentamicin
2 ☐ allergy to penicillin G
3 ☐ development of heat rash

A ☐ 1, 2, 3
B ☐ 1, 2 only
C ☐ 2, 3 only
D ☐ 1 only
E ☐ 3 only

Q63 Manifestations of bacterial endocarditis include:

1 ☐ prolonged fever
2 ☐ embolic phenomena
3 ☐ renal failure

A ☐ 1, 2, 3
B ☐ 1, 2 only
C ☐ 2, 3 only
D ☐ 1 only
E ☐ 3 only

Questions 64–74 involve the following case:

JZ is a 78-year-old obese male who is diagnosed with an acute attack of gout.

PMH hypertension, heart failure
DH enalapril tablets 5 mg daily
  atenolol tablets 100 mg daily
  bendroflumethiazide tablets 5 mg daily
  aspirin ec tablets 75 mg daily

He is started on colchicine tablets 500 µg twice daily for six days.

Q64 Gout:

A ☐ may be due to excessive production of uric acid
B ☐ may be due to increased renal elimination of uric acid
C ☐ results in the deposition of crystals of xanthine in the joints
D ☐ is characterised by excessive calcium deposited in the joints
E ☐ is the result of hypouricaemia

Q65 Gout may be precipitated in JZ by:

1 ☐ heart failure
2 ☐ bendroflumethiazide
3 ☐ excessive consumption of meat in the diet

A ☐ 1, 2, 3
B ☐ 1, 2 only
C ☐ 2, 3 only
D ☐ 1 only
E ☐ 3 only

Q66   Gout:

1   ☐   presents as a painful condition in the big toe
2   ☐   onset is insidious
3   ☐   recurrence is rare

A   ☐   1, 2, 3
B   ☐   1, 2 only
C   ☐   2, 3 only
D   ☐   1 only
E   ☐   3 only

Q67   Diagnosis of gout:

1   ☐   is based on clinical signs
2   ☐   requires confirmation of urate crystals in the synovial fluid of affected joint
3   ☐   requires a positive ESR level

A   ☐   1, 2, 3
B   ☐   1, 2 only
C   ☐   2, 3 only
D   ☐   1 only
E   ☐   3 only

Q68   Non-pharmacological measures for JZ include:

1   ☐   resting the affected joint
2   ☐   maintaining a high fluid intake
3   ☐   maintaining a high calcium intake

A   ☐   1, 2, 3
B   ☐   1, 2 only
C   ☐   2, 3 only
D   ☐   1 only
E   ☐   3 only

Q69   Colchicine:

1   ❑ reduces the inflammatory reaction to urate crystals
2   ❑ provides dramatic relief from acute attacks of gout
3   ❑ is also used in rheumatoid arthritis

A   ❑ 1, 2, 3
B   ❑ 1, 2 only
C   ❑ 2, 3 only
D   ❑ 1 only
E   ❑ 3 only

Q70   Colchicine:

1   ❑ should be used when there is a contraindication to NSAIDs
2   ❑ is more toxic than NSAIDs
3   ❑ occurrence of diarrhoea and vomiting are used as an index
      to review therapy

A   ❑ 1, 2, 3
B   ❑ 1, 2 only
C   ❑ 2, 3 only
D   ❑ 1 only
E   ❑ 3 only

Q71   Alternatives to colchicine in the management of gout include:

1   ❑ indometacin
2   ❑ diclofenac
3   ❑ aspirin

A   ❑ 1, 2, 3
B   ❑ 1, 2 only
C   ❑ 2, 3 only
D   ❑ 1 only
E   ❑ 3 only

Q72   To prevent further attacks, JZ should be advised to:

1   ❑ lose weight
2   ❑ follow a diet low in purines
3   ❑ keep taking colchicine on a long-term basis

A   ❑ 1, 2, 3
B   ❑ 1, 2 only
C   ❑ 2, 3 only
D   ❑ 1 only
E   ❑ 3 only

Q73   Allopurinol:

1   ❑ should be started 2–3 weeks after the acute attack has subsided
2   ❑ reduces urate production
3   ❑ is given once daily

A   ❑ 1, 2, 3
B   ❑ 1, 2 only
C   ❑ 2, 3 only
D   ❑ 1 only
E   ❑ 3 only

Q74   Uricosuric agents:

1   ❑ can be used instead of allopurinol
2   ❑ are ineffective in patients with impaired renal function
3   ❑ increase renal urate excretion

A   ❑ 1, 2, 3
B   ❑ 1, 2 only
C   ❑ 2, 3 only
D   ❑ 1 only
E   ❑ 3 only

Questions 75–80 involve the following case:

HG is a 71-year-old female with a history of Sjögren's syndrome. She presents with complaints of dry eyes and dry mouth.

At the time the patient was on aspirin 150 mg daily, dipyridamole 25 mg tds, glimepiride 1 mg daily and atenolol 100 mg daily. Recently hypothyroidism was diagnosed and she was started on thyroxine 50 µg daily. During a recent follow up, her diabetologist added metformin 500 mg daily because her blood glucose level was 13.8 mmol/l. She was also started on simvastatin 10 mg nocte.

Her ESR is 109 mm/h and she has a positive rheumatoid factor.

Methylcellulose eye drops to be used as required are recommended to HG.

Q75 In view of the recent amendments to her treatment, HG should be advised to:

1 ☐ take thyroxine tablet in the morning
2 ☐ take metformin tablet with food
3 ☐ take dipyridamole tablets before food

A ☐ 1, 2, 3
B ☐ 1, 2 only
C ☐ 2, 3 only
D ☐ 1 only
E ☐ 3 only

Q76 Hypothyroidism:

1 ☐ may have an insidious onset in the elderly
2 ☐ may cause dry eyes
3 ☐ may induce hypoglycaemia

A   ☐ 1, 2, 3
B   ☐ 1, 2 only
C   ☐ 2, 3 only
D   ☐ 1 only
E   ☐ 3 only

Q77   Drugs that could significantly interact with thyroxine include:

1   ☐ warfarin
2   ☐ simvastatin
3   ☐ ranitidine

A   ☐ 1, 2, 3
B   ☐ 1, 2 only
C   ☐ 2, 3 only
D   ☐ 1 only
E   ☐ 3 only

Q78   Caution should be undertaken when starting thyroxine in:

1   ☐ elderly patients
2   ☐ diabetics
3   ☐ patients with cardiovascular disorders

A   ☐ 1, 2, 3
B   ☐ 1, 2 only
C   ☐ 2, 3 only
D   ☐ 1 only
E   ☐ 3 only

Q79   Side-effects associated with thyroxine include:

1   ❑ diarrhoea
2   ❑ anginal pain
3   ❑ bradycardia

A   ❑ 1, 2, 3
B   ❑ 1, 2 only
C   ❑ 2, 3 only
D   ❑ 1 only
E   ❑ 3 only

Q80   Total thyroid hormones:

1   ❑ concentration in plasma changes with alterations in the amount of thyroxine-binding globulin in plasma
2   ❑ concentration is used as the main diagnostic marker for hypothyroidism
3   ❑ act as antibodies to thyroglobulin

A   ❑ 1, 2, 3
B   ❑ 1, 2 only
C   ❑ 2, 3 only
D   ❑ 1 only
E   ❑ 3 only

Test 1

Answers

Questions 1–3

Interpretation of clinical laboratory tests is useful during diagnosis and during therapeutic monitoring. Common laboratory tests include electrolytes, haematology, renal function tests and liver function tests. In interpreting clinical laboratory tests, it is important to use different tests to corroborate information because laboratory errors are not uncommon, caused by, for example, spoiled specimens, incorrect amount of specimen and medications that could interfere with test results. Furthermore, laboratory investigations are best collaborated through supporting clinical evidence. When possible laboratory results are best evaluated in an holistic approach.

A1   A

The mean corpuscular haemoglobin concentration (MCHC) is a red cell index that forms part of haematology tests. It measures the average concentration of haemoglobin in erythrocytes (red blood cells). It is decreased in different presentations of anaemia, including iron deficiency anaemia and in thalassemia. In iron deficiency anaemia, the haematocrit value (space occupied by packed erythrocytes) is decreased.

A2   B

The measurement of total and differential white blood cell (WBC) count is a part of all routine laboratory diagnostic evaluations. It is helpful in the evaluation of a patient with an infection, although a high WBC count may also be found in other conditions such as neoplasma, allergy and immunosuppression. One type of WBCs is the lymphocytes, their primary function being to fight chronic bacterial infection and acute viral infections. Lymphocytes can be further classified into B cells and T cells. The mature B cells produce immuno-globulins. The T cells have cell-mediated immunity as a major property, where they act directly to eliminate certain microorganisms and regulate the activity of B cells in producing immunoglobulins. An increased number of lymphocytes (lymphocytosis) occurs with viral infections, such as in patients with upper respiratory tract infections, mumps and infectious mononucleosis.

A3   E

Thrombocytes (platelets) are elements in blood, their main role being the maintenance of vascular integrity. In idiopathic thrombocytopenia purpura there is a deficiency of platelets leading to bruising and bleeding. Idiopathic thrombocytopenia purpura is associated with the occurrence of antibodies to platelets.

Questions 4–6

When approaching therapeutic management of a patient, it is essential to familiarise yourself with background information on the disease state(s) and on the patient's presenting complaints.

A4   D

Myopathy is a condition affecting the skeletal muscle, and which is manifested by muscle weakness and wasting. Histological changes occur in the muscle tissues, similar to those that occur in muscular dystrophies.

A5   A

Tachypnoea is an abnormally fast breathing rate. It is characteristic of respiratory diseases and occurs in hyperpyrexia. It occurs as a result of over-activity at the level of the sympathetic nervous system.

A6   E

Dysphasia (aphasia) is a condition resulting in impairment of the language aspect of speech. It usually occurs as a result of cerebral cortex injury, such as after surgery for a brain tumour or after a cerebral stroke. The presence of dysphasia is frequently accompanied by writing disorders.

Questions 7–26

A7   D

Prednisolone is a corticosteroid with a predominantly glucocorticoid activity. However, owing to minor mineralcorticoid activity, it may still cause electrolyte imbalance, namely sodium and water retention and potassium loss. Salbutamol and propranolol do not interfere with plasma sodium electrolyte levels. Salbutamol may precipitate hypokalaemia, especially with parenteral administration or after nebulisation. The risk of hypokalaemia with salbutamol therapy may be increased with concomitant administration of certain drugs, such as corticosteroids and diuretics.

A8   A

Paget's disease, neuropathy and haemophilia are all conditions that are associated with the occurrence of muscular or joint pain. Paget's disease is a disease of the bone where there is excessive bone destruction and abnormalities in bone repair. The condition may be associated with bone pain, bone deformity, fractures and pain caused by pressure on nerves. However, Paget's disease may be asymptomatic. Neuropathy is a condition where there is inflammation or degeneration of the peripheral nerves. It may occur as a complication of long-standing uncontrolled diabetes. Patients complain of excruciating pain in the peripheries. In haemophilia there is a deficiency of one of the factors necessary for blood coagulation. Patients with haemophilia are prone to develop bleeding in joints, resulting in pain.

A9   A

Several persistent unexplained symptoms may indicate neoplastic disease and would require further assessment to understand the underlying pathology. Symptoms such as skin ulceration, unexplained fractures and general debility may indicate neoplastic disease. Skin ulceration could occur as a result of skin carcinoma. Unexplained fractures may be due to carcinoma involving the bone structure. This tumour usually occurs as a secondary tumour to a solid tumour that has originated in another area. General debility may be a characteristic of malignant disorders, such as chronic myelocytic leukaemia, Hodgkin's disease, non-Hodgkin's lymphoma and various solid tumours.

A10   C

The administration of cytotoxic chemotherapy regimen may fail to achieve remission in an individual patient compared with a cohort of patients owing to drug resistance. Tumour cells may be inherently resistant or acquire resistance after a number of treatment sessions. Tumour cell resistance may be explained by a reduction of intracellular drug concentration, enzymatic deactivation of the drug, and by increased repair of damaged DNA. If the drugs fail to penetrate the solid tumour, then they are not in a position to achieve cell death.

A11   B

In Parkinson's disease patients have problems with postural stability, movement and verbal communication. The involvement of physiotherapists and speech therapists helps the patient to cope with the loss of mobility, to retain activity as much as possible and to keep communication with carers. Patients with Parkinson's disease have a mask-like expression, a monotonous voice and may experience fatigue, drooling of saliva, dysphagia, constipation, excessive swelling, speech and depressive disorders. Severe chronic pain is not a presentation that is related to the occurrence of Parkinson's disease.

A12 B

Ultrasound scanning is a non-invasive, non-toxic diagnostic procedure that can be used to examine internal organs. It does not involve radiation. It is based on sound waves that travel through the body tissues at different speed depending on the density and elasticity of the organ tissues. Ultrasound scanning is used to diagnose conditions such as tumours in areas such as abdomen, heart, liver and kidneys. It is also used to assess the development of the fetus.

A13 B

Creatinine clearance is the rate of removal of creatinine from the body by the kidney during glomerular filtration. It gives a measure of the glomerular filtration rate (GFR). The measured creatinine clearance is more accurate in the assessment of renal function compared with the calculated creatinine clearance, which is based on a formula where the serum creatinine concentration is used. To measure the creatinine clearance, a 24-h urine collection and a serum sample are required.

A14 D

Isosorbide dinitrate is a nitrate that is a more stable preparation compared with glyceryl trinitrate. Isosorbide dinitrate tablets are stable and do not require special storage conditions. It is used in the prophylaxis and treatment of angina and in left ventricular failure. The most common side-effect that may occur is throbbing headache. Occurrence of this side-effect usually decreases after a few days. The headache is associated with peripheral vasodilation. Tolerance to the peripheral effects occurs early on in treatment.

A15 B

Adrenaline is a potent sympathomimetic agent that is used in cardiac arrest by intravenous injection preferably through a central line. It is the first-line treatment in anaphylaxis, where it is usually given intramuscularly. Stimulation of the alpha-adrenergic receptors produces vasoconstriction that may result in hypertension. Blood pressure should be monitored during administration of adrenaline. It should be used with caution in patients with hypertension. Over-dosage may cause a sharp rise in blood pressure.

A16   C

Methadone is an opioid agonist that is itself addictive and is used in the management of patients who are physically dependent on opioids. Its advantage in the management of opioid dependence is that it is administered as a single daily dose, usually as an oral solution.

A17   A

Tamoxifen is an oestrogen-receptor antagonist that is used for breast cancer and anovulatory infertility. Its side-effects are very similar to the menopausal phase and hot flushes are a common side-effect. Suppression of menstruation may occur in premenopausal women. As the use of tamoxifen is associated with an increased risk of endometrial changes, including hyperplasia, polyps, cancer and uterine sarcoma, occurrence of menstrual abnormalities, including abnormal vaginal bleeding and vaginal discharge, warrant immediate investi-gation. Hence patients receiving tamoxifen should be advised that if menstrual irregularities occur they should seek medical advice. Tamoxifen can increase the risk of thromboembolism, and therefore patients should be advised about the symptoms that may indicate onset of thromboembolism, such as sudden breathlessness and pain in the calf, so that they seek advice immediately.

A18   B

Sodium bicarbonate as a parenteral preparation for fluid and electrolyte imbalance is used in severe metabolic acidosis, for example, in renal failure when blood pH is less than 7.1. By administering sodium bicarbonate, in conjunction with sodium chloride when there is also sodium depletion, pH of blood is increased. Sodium bicarbonate may also alkalinise the urine, which will increase the excretion of weak acids. In hypomagnesaemia, magnesium sulphate intravenous infusion is administered.

A19   A

Phytomenadione is vitamin K1. Vitamin K is a fat-soluble vitamin that is required for the hepatic synthesis of prothrombin and other blood clotting factors (factors VII, IX, X and proteins C and S). Neonates are particularly prone to develop vitamin K deficiency and this may lead to haemorrhagic disease including intracranial bleeding. It may be used in babies at birth as a single intramuscular injection to prevent vitamin K deficiency bleeding. Vitamin K deficiency may occur in underweight neonates owing to inadequate synthesis.

A20   A

Enoxaparin is a low-molecular-weight heparin that has a longer duration of action when compared with unfractionated heparin. The dose for enoxaparin varies from the dose for heparin; for example, in the prophylaxis of deep vein thrombosis before surgery, 2000 units of enoxaparin are administered 2 hours before surgery, whereas for heparin 5000 units are administered 2 hours before surgery. As with heparin, thrombocytopenia may occur with the administration of low molecular weight heparins. Enoxaparin should be avoided in patients who have developed thrombocytopenia with heparin. Regular monitoring is required when the patient is also taking any drugs that interfere with haemostasis. The use of oral anticoagulants, dipyridamole, aspirin and other non-steroidal anti-inflammatory drugs (NSAIDs) should be reviewed. Care should be taken when used in conjunction with thrombolytic enzymes and high doses of penicillins and cephalosporins.

A21   A

Isotretinoin is a retinoid that may be used orally in the specialist management of severe acne vulgaris. Retinoids have many contraindications and serious side-effects. Isotretinoin is teratogenic and therefore women of child-bearing age should be advised to avoid pregnancy and to practise effective contraception. Retinoids should only be used in premenopausal women if they have severe disabling skin disease that is resistant to other treatment and if pregnancy has been excluded. Treatment with oral isotretinoin should be started only during the second or third day of a menstrual cycle and contraceptive precautions should be continued for at least 4 weeks after the end of treatment. Common side-effects of oral isotretinoin treatment include dryness of the skin presenting with dermatitis, scaling, thinning, erythema and pruritus, epidermal fragility and dryness of the lips, pharyngeal mucosa and nasal mucosa. During treatment and for at least 6 months from stopping treatment, patients should be advised to avoid wax epilation because of a risk of epidermal stripping, and to avoid dermabrasion and laser skin treatment as there is risk of scarring. Patients should be advised to avoid exposure to ultraviolet light and to use sunscreens, emollients and lip balms regularly during treatment.

A22   C

Colonoscopy is a diagnostic procedure that is carried out to examine the colon and terminal ileum. To aid the direct observation of the bowel, bowel cleansing is required before the procedure. Patients are advised to follow a clear-liquid diet before the procedure at least for one day. Bowel cleansing preparations containing magnesium salts are administered orally on the day before the procedure. They produce rapid evacuation of the bowels. Patient should not consume any food or fluids from 6–8 hours before the procedure.

A23   B

Patients with a history of asthma presenting with a chest infection should be referred for assessment about the need to use antibacterial agents and the necessity of reviewing asthma treatment. A paediatric patient is at a higher risk of rapid deterioration. Patients who are using diuretics are more prone to dehydration in a hot climate. If they present symptoms of a heat stroke they should be referred for assessment of their medical condition, as they are at higher risk of developing complications. Acute diarrhoea may be treated by recommending oral rehydration salts. The patient is asked to contact a pharmacist, should the situation get worse or if it is not managed within a few days.

A24   B

Helicobacter pylori, a Gram-negative bacterium, is implicated as a cause of chronic gastritis and peptic ulceration. Its eradication in the stomach entails a triple-therapy regimen that is based on a proton pump inhibitor such as omeprazole, and two anti-infective agents, namely amoxicillin and either clarithromycin or metronidazole. In patients who are penicillin sensitive, the triple therapy regimen considered consists of a proton pump inhibitor, clarithromycin and metronidazole. Telithromycin is a derivative of erythromycin that is not used in *Helicobacter pylori* eradication therapy.

A25   D

In patients affected by the human immunodeficiency virus (HIV), the aim of treatment is to decrease the plasma viral load as much as possible for the longest possible time. Before starting treatment or when changing drug therapy, viral sensitivity to antiretroviral agents should be established. The onset of drug resistance is reduced by using combination of drugs so as to have a synergistic or additive effect. Care should be taken to ensure that the combination used does not have an additive toxicity as antiretrovirals are toxic. Common combinations include two nucleoside reverse transcriptase inhibitors and either an HIV-protease inhibitor or a non-nucleoside reverse transcriptase inhibitor. In HIV, viral replication leading to accumulation of mutations results in the emergence of drug-resistant variants and consequently disease progression.

A26   B

Diabetic ketoacidosis is a condition where there is acidosis and an accumulation of ketones in the body resulting from extensive breakdown of fat. It occurs in patients with hyperglycaemia and ketosis as a result of insulin deficiency. Normally diabetic patients with hyperglycaemia do not progress to diabetic ketoacidosis. Factors that could precipitate the condition include infection, dehydration, surgery, sustained strenuous exercise, trauma. Patients with diabetic ketoacidosis present with a fruity odour of acetone on the breath, mental confusion, dyspnoea, nausea, vomiting, and dehydration. The condition may lead to coma. Retinopathy is a complication of diabetes that could lead to blindness.

Questions 27–31

Pulmonary oedema may result from the failure of a number of homeostatic mechanisms and it is a condition that can develop acutely and can be fatal. It most commonly occurs as a result of chronic heart failure. Diuretics provide a dramatic improvement of the condition.

A27   C

Signs and symptoms of pulmonary oedema include dyspnoea, cough, orthopnoea, and tachypnoea. Owing to the accumulation of extravascular fluid in lung tissues, alveoli and in the extremities, the patient may present with an increase in weight.

A28   C

An acute attack of pulmonary oedema may develop due to progressive heart failure or when the patient is not compliant with medication, particularly the diuretic therapy. It may also occur due to hypervolaemia, such as when compromised and non-compromised patients are exposed to an excessive fluid infusion rate or to a high sodium intake. Conditions that lead to an increased metabolic demand, such as high fever and hyperthyroidism, may also precipitate acute pulmonary oedema.

A29   B

Metolazone is a diuretic that is associated with profound diuresis, especially when it is combined with a loop diuretic. Patients receiving metolazone should be monitored for electrolyte imbalance and outcome of therapy may be assessed by measuring change in body weight and urine production.

A30   A

Metolazone is a diuretic with actions similar to a thiazide diuretic, and bumetanide is a loop diuretic. Metolazone has a long duration of action of about 12–24 h compared with intravenous bumetanide, which has a duration of action of 0.5–1 h. Diuretics increase diuresis and result in a reduction of blood volume.

A31   B

Once PS is stabilised, a long-term therapeutic plan should be carried out. Metolazone treatment should be withdrawn, after which a change from bumetanide to oral therapy should be attempted. The patient should be advised about the importance of compliance with bumetanide, and that the unwanted effect of increased diuresis with oral treatment usually decreases with time. The patient should be advised to take the drug in the morning. Potassium levels should be monitored and, if the patient is not taking any drugs with a potassium-sparing effect, then potassium supplements should be considered when bumetanide therapy is given long-term.

Questions 32–38

CA is a diabetic patient whose blood glucose level needs monitoring. Upon discharge the pharmacist needs to advise the patient on her condition and on her medication so as to avoid future deterioration. She is showing signs of dehydration and uncontrolled blood glucose levels.

A32   B

Rehydration and control of hyperglycaemia are the primary aims. Her skin condition is a secondary complication of uncontrolled diabetes. The antibacterial agent is continued and patient is started on an antidiabetic drug (glibenclamide) to control blood glucose levels. CA is also administered haloperidol (an antipsychotic).

A33   B

In patients who are dehydrated, urine output is very much decreased. The extent of rehydration, which is being undertaken using intravenous infusion of sodium chloride, should be assessed by monitoring urine output. Regular blood glucose monitoring is required and, if necessary, antidiabetic therapy should be reviewed.

A34   B

Clinical features of hyperglycaemia include thirst, dry mouth, reduced skin turgor, polyuria, nocturia. A diabetic complication is an increased susceptibility to infection especially in the skin, vaginal area and peripheries.

A35   C

Ciprofloxacin may be administered at a dose of 500 mg orally twice daily. As CA has been started on this antibacterial agent only the day before her admission, there is no indication that warrants a need to increase the dose or review the therapy because the drug is ineffective. The sodium chloride infusion is required to rehydrate the patient, and should be continued until normal urine flow is achieved. The pharmacist could monitor the patient's progress and advise the prescribing team when to withdraw the infusion. There is no apparent rationale for the use of haloperidol in this elderly patient. Her state of confusion is due to her hyperglycaemic state, which has precipitated dehydration. Correction of these complications should improve her confusion. Haloperidol has a rapid effect on hyperactive states and initial doses may help to calm down the patient. However, continued use may precipitate hypo-glycaemia. Continued treatment with haloperidol should be reviewed.

A36   A

Glibenclamide and gliclazide are oral sulphonylureas that are used in diabetes to augment secretion of insulin. They are effective only in patients with residual pancreatic beta-cell activity. Gliclazide is a shorter-acting product. It has a duration of action of about 12 h whereas glibenclamide has a duration of action of up to 24 h. The shorter-acting product is less likely to cause hypoglycaemia. CA is an elderly patient, who may present with a slower metabolism of the drug; she may be living alone and may have problems with maintaining regular meals. The dose of glibenclamide for elderly patients is usually 2.5 mg after breakfast.

A37   B

CA should be advised to consume small, frequent regular meals that are low in fat and carbohydrate content. She should be educated on the foods to include in her diet and about the importance of having a regular schedule of food intake to avoid hypoglycaemic attacks. She should be reminded that she has to continue taking the glibenclamide tablet daily at breakfast to avoid recurrence of hyperglycaemia.

A38   E

Hypoglycaemia with sulphonylureas may occur either because of excessive doses or skipped meals. If CA continues to take her glibenclamide tablets and she skips meals, there is a higher risk of hypoglycaemia.

Questions 39–41

Alcohol is a central nervous system depressant. Conditions that are associated with alcoholism include liver disease, cardiomyopathy, pancreatitis and gastrointestinal disease. Signs and symptoms of alcohol withdrawal include tremor, tachycardia, diaphoresis, labile blood pressure, anxiety, nausea and vomiting, hallucinations and seizures.

A39   A

Promethazine is a sedating antihistamine, which BD was probably using initially for the insomnia and sleep disorders that are associated with alcohol withdrawal syndrome. Side-effects that could occur with the use of promethazine, especially in overdosage include drowsiness, headache, and antimuscarinic effects such as blurred vision and urinary retention.

A40   C

Promethazine is a sedating antihistamine that could be used in the symptomatic relief of allergy of nasal or dermatological origin, as a hypnotic and in motion sickness. It can be used in adults and children over 2 years.

A41   D

Long-acting benzodiazepines such as diazepam could be used in alcohol withdrawal to counteract the withdrawal symptoms. In alcohol withdrawal, symptoms of the initial phases do not necessarily diminish as withdrawal advances. This depends on the amount of alcohol consumed, on the abruptness of discontinuation and on the patient's general well-being. When the patient is started on a benzodiazepine, advice on alcohol abstinence should be provided. Also the patient should be referred to patient-support groups, to provide the necessary psychosocial support for the management of alcohol abuse.

Questions 42–44

A myocardial infarction, also referred to as a heart attack, is the necrosis of a portion of the cardiac muscle and occurs due to occlusion of the coronary artery, either because of atherosclerosis or thrombus or a spasm. The patient presents with a crushing chest pain that may radiate to the left arm, neck and epigastrium. Statins are used as lipid-lowering agents in conjunction with diet to reduce total cholesterol and low-density-lipoprotein cholesterol as a secondary prevention of the recurrence of cardiovascular disease. They reduce morbidity and mortality in these patients.

A42   B

Simvastatin is a statin and it may cause rare but significant side-effects of myalgia, myositis and myopathy. Patient should be advised to report any muscle pain, tenderness and weakness as they could be signs of these side-effects. Higher efficacy has been shown with the administration of simvastatin at night, compared with in the morning, probably because cholesterol bio-synthesis reaches a peak during the night.

A43   A

Common side-effects associated with statins include headache, gastrointestinal symptoms and altered liver function tests.

A44 B

The use of lipid-regulating drugs, including statins, should be combined with a low-fat diet and moderate exercise such as walking so as to reduce the risk of cardiovascular disease.

Questions 45–47

Medication review, particularly for elderly patients, is useful to evaluate rationale for drug therapy, to monitor outcomes, to identify problems with the medications and to re-inforce patient counselling. GD is receiving dipyridamole and aspirin as antiplatelet drugs; timotol, a beta-blocker; and lactulose, an osmotic laxative.

A45 C

Dipyridamole is used as an oral preparation for the prophylaxis of thromboembolism and for the secondary prevention of ischaemic stroke and transient ischaemic attacks. It may cause increased bleeding during or after surgery and it may induce bleeding in patients receiving oral anticoagulants without altering the prothrombin time. It may be used in combination with low-dose aspirin as this combination may further reduce the risk of ischaemia.

A46 E

Lactulose is a semi-synthetic disaccharide that can be safely used on a long-term basis in elderly patients to maintain regular bowel evacuation, especially in patients with limited mobility. The initial adult dose of lactulose is 15 ml twice daily and this may be adjusted according to the individual's needs. Therefore 20 ml daily dose is an acceptable dosage regimen.

A47   D

GD is receiving prophylactic therapy for secondary prevention of cerebro-vascular and cardiovascular disease, timotol for glaucoma and lactulose to maintain regular bowel movements.

Questions 48–53

SP is presenting with a deterioration of congestive heart failure presenting mainly as oedema. Management of congestive heart failure may include an angiotensin-converting enzyme inhibitor (ACE) such as enalapril, a diuretic if there is fluid overload, spironolactone, beta-blockers and digoxin.

A48   B

SP is presenting the classic symptoms of heart failure, namely tiredness, shortness of breath and oedema. In SP the aims are to control the symptoms of heart failure and limit the deterioration of the condition leading to oedema.

A49   A

Spironolactone is a potassium-sparing diuretic that acts by antagonising aldos-terone. It can be used in patients already receiving an ACE inhibitor to reduce the symptoms and mortality associated with congestive heart failure. Low doses of spironolactone are used and the maximum dose is 25 mg daily.

A50   B

In patients with congestive heart failure receiving spironolactone, the moni-toring of serum creatinine and potassium is necessary. Spironolactone should not be used in patients with hyperkalaemia or in severe renal impairment.

A51 A

Losartan is an angiotensin-II receptor antagonist which may be used as an alternative to ACE inhibitors in patients who develop cough. The usual maintenance dose for losartan is 50 mg daily.

A52 C

Digoxin is a cardiac glycoside that may be used in patients with heart failure when there is atrial fibrillation. It is a positive inotropic drug and it increases contractility of the heart thus increasing cardiac output. It has a long halflife.

A53 B

Digoxin has a narrow therapeutic margin and treatment may lead to digitalis toxicity, which may be manifested by nausea, vomiting, anorexia, diarrhoea and abdominal pain. This may progress to cardiac toxicity resulting in heart block. Hypokalaemia in patients receiving digoxin increases risk of digitalis toxicity. It is necessary to monitor plasma potassium levels and plasma digoxin concentrations. In patients who are already receiving spironolactone or an ACE inhibitor, risk of hypokalaemia is minimal.

Questions 54–57

LB has herpes zoster infection, also known as shingles. Antiviral treatment reduces the severity and duration of pain, reduces complications and reduces viral shedding. Complications of shingles include postherpetic neuralgia which lasts months to years, eye or ear involvement. Treatment with antiviral drugs should be started within 72 h of the onset of the rash.

A54   B

LB has herpes zoster infection. It is an acute infection due to re-activation of the varicella zoster virus which is latent in the body. It affects mainly adults and is characterised by the development of painful vesicles that follow the underlying route of a nerve. The vesicles are usually unilaterally distributed over the body.

A55   B

The patient should be advised to take aciclovir tablets at regular intervals and to complete the prescribed course. The patient should be advised to avoid exposure to sunlight, as aciclovir may cause photosensitivity.

A56   A

Gastrointestinal side-effects of aciclovir include nausea, vomiting, abdominal pain and diarrhoea. Other side-effects are headache, fatigue, rash, urticaria and pruritus.

A57   B

Calamine lotion may be used by LB to reduce itching and to provide symptomatic relief of the pain. Amitriptyline may be used as an adjuvant analgesic, particularly if the patient develops postherpetic neuralgia. In addition an analgesic such as a non-steroidal product and a topical corticosteroid to reduce severe inflammation may be considered.

Questions 58–63

Bacterial endocarditis is an infective condition affecting the endocardium and the cardiac valves. It is more common when there are cardiac abnormalities such as aortic valve disease, pulmonary stenosis and mitral stenosis or in the presence of prosthetic valves. In infective endocarditis, it is essential to identify causative organism, to eradicate the organism and to prevent recurrence of infection. It usually occurs when bacteria are released from an infected site such as a tooth or skin abscess or after a surgical intervention.

A58   B

Benzylpenicillin is Penicillin G.

A59   D

Each vial contains 0.6 g and therefore for a dose of 1.8 g, three vials are required.

A60   C

Penicillin G, as with all penicillins, is a bactericidal and acts by interfering with bacterial cell-wall synthesis. Penicillin G is inactivated by bacterial beta-lactamases. As it is inactivated by gastric acid, and absorption from the gut is very low, it is administered as an intramuscular injection or by slow intravenous injection or by infusion.

A61   D

Gentamicin is an aminoglycoside that has a bactericidal action against Gram-negative and Gram-positive bacteria. It is excreted primarily by the kidneys, so in renal impairment, the dose should be reduced or the dosing intervals increased. Aminoglycosides are not absorbed from the gastrointestinal tract, and therefore for a systemic effect, parenteral administration is required.

A62   A

Hypersensitivity to antibacterial agents and the development of a heat rash are possible.

A63   A

The clinical presentation of bacterial endocarditis varies. Usually there is an insidious onset and the patient's condition starts to deteriorate gradually. Fever is the most common finding, usually occurring at a relatively low grade. Initial symptoms are fatigue, low-grade fever, weakness, anorexia and weight loss. Embolic phenomena such as splenic or renal infarction and skin manifestations occur in a large number of cases. Peripheral manifestations of endocarditis may occur, such as petechiae and finger clubbing. In some patients signs of renal failure are also manifested.

Questions 64–74

JZ presents with an acute attack of gout. He is on medication to control his hypertension and heart failure. He is taking an angiotensin-converting enzyme inhibitor (enalapril), a beta-adrenoceptor blocker (atenolol), a thiazide diuretic (bendroflumethiazide) and aspirin as an antiplatelet agent to prevent occurrence of cerebrovascular disease and myocardial infarction.

A64   A

Gout is a condition associated with either an increased production of uric acid or a decreased excretion of uric acid. Excess uric acid in the body is converted to sodium urate crystals that are deposited in joints, most commonly in the big toe. Increased levels of serum uric acid may be due to excessive production of uric acid or to excessive destruction of cells and therefore breakdown of nucleic acids, resulting in the production of uric acid.

A65   A

Heart failure is a condition that may increase risk of hyperuricaemia. Diuretics interfere with the excretion of uric acid and alter the concentration of uric acid in blood. This results in precipitation of uric acid salts from the blood which become deposited in the joints. A diet that consists of excessive consumption of purine-rich food such as meat and organ meat increases production of uric acid.

A66   D

An acute attack of gout is characterised by a rapid onset of pain, swelling and inflammation usually affecting the first metatarsophalangeal joint in the big toe. Initially, the attack is monoarticular but it may progress to include other joints. Attacks could recur with no clear provocation.

A67   D

The clinical signs are so characteristic of the condition that diagnosis could be based on their presentation. Concentration of urate crystals in the synovial fluid of joints correlates very closely with serum levels. Serum uric acid levels may be measured, particulary to monitor treatment. Hyperuricaemia also tends to be present in other arthritic disease states. The erythrocyte sedimentation rate (ESR) is a non-specific test that indicates occurrence of infection or inflammatory diseases. As it is a non-specific test, its relevance to the diagnosis of gout is minimal.

A68   B

JZ should be advised to rest the affected joint, maintain good fluid intake and to take the prescribed drug. The use of colchicine in older people may precipitate dehydration and electrolyte imbalance because of the common occurrence of nausea, vomiting and diarrhoea as side-effects. JZ should be advised to report side-effects immediately.

A69   B

Colchicine is an effective drug, which is used in the acute management of gout or for short-term prophylaxis during initial therapy with allopurinol or other uricosuric agents. Its use is limited by the occurrence of side-effects, especially at high doses or in patients with renal or hepatic disease. It produces a dramatic response in acute gout probably by acting as an antimitotic and inhibiting leucocyte mobility to the inflamed areas.

A70   A

Usually non-steroidal anti-inflammatory drugs are used as first-line treatment in the management of acute attacks of gout. They counteract the pain and reduce the inflammation. JZ suffers from heart failure and colchicine is preferred to avoid the fluid retention that may occur with NSAIDs. Also, NSAIDs may interact with the medications that JZ is taking, namely the diuretics and anti-hypertensive agents, causing a decrease in the hypotensive effect. Although this interaction is usually not of clinical significance, it is worth considering other therapeutic options. The disadvantage of colchicine is that it is commonly associated with side-effects, particularly signs of gastrointestinal toxicity manifested as diarrhoea and vomiting. Occurrence of these side-effects indicates that the dose should be reviewed. Colchicine is associated with cumulative toxicity and diarrhoea, nausea, vomiting and abdominal pain are the first signs of toxicity. The dose should be stopped or reduced depending on the patient's symptoms.

A71   B

Non-steroidal drugs such as indometacin and diclofenac are considered in the management of acute attacks of gout. Aspirin and its derivatives should be avoided during an acute attack as these agents compete with uric acid for excretion and may worsen rather than decrease the symptoms. In fact it is worth considering stopping the aspirin 75 mg daily dose until the acute attack subsides. The dose is relatively low but the patient already has other factors that may be contributing to the condition and the aspirin is used as a prophylactic agent in JZ.

A72   B

Obesity, heart failure and drug therapy are all factors in JZ which increase susceptibility to gout. JZ should be advised on how to counteract the factors that may be corrected. He should be advised to lose weight, which will help him to manage his cardiovascular risk better, as well as to decrease the recurrence of gout. He should be advised to take regular exercise that is not very strenuous, such as short walks and to follow a healthy diet that is based on fruit and vegetables, which will be low in purines.

A73   A

Allopurinol is used for the long-term prophylaxis of gout and is considered for patients who have a high incidence of recurrence. It reduces uric acid production by inhibiting the enzyme xanthine oxidase, which brings about the oxidation of hypoxanthine to xanthine and of xanthine to uric acid. As allopurinol may prolong an attack or precipitate it, it should not be started during an acute attack. It should be started 2–3 weeks after the acute attack has subsided. It is given in a once-daily dose. It has an active metabolite, oxipurinol, which has a plasma halflife of 15 or more hours.

A74   A

Uricosuric drugs include sulfinpyrazone and probenecid. Like allopurinol, they may be used as prophylactic agents. They should be avoided in patients with overproduction of uric acid and are ineffective in patients with poor renal function. They inhibit the renal tubular re-absorption of uric acid and therefore increase urinary excretion of uric acid. Patients should be advised to consume a good fluid intake of at least two litres a day. This will decrease the risk of uric acid stone formation.

Questions 75–80

HG suffers from Sjögren's syndrome, a condition that is frequently associated with rheumatoid arthritis and Raynaud's phenomenon. The condition presents with a deficient moisture production of the lacrimal, salivary and other glands resulting in dryness of the mouth, eyes and other mucous membranes. The patient may also have the classic characteristics of rheumatoid arthritis. HG is a diabetic and is taking a sulphonylurea (glimepiride) and a biguanide (metformin). She is on a beta-blocker (atenolol) and an antiplatelet drug (dipyridamole) indicating possibility of a history of cardiovascular disease. She is taking simvastatin as a lipid-regulating drug. HG has recently been diagnosed with hypothyroidism and she was prescribed thyroxine. Her ESR is elevated (>30 mm/h) and she is seropositive for rheumatoid factor.

A75   A

Thyroxine, levothyroxine, is a thyroid hormone used in hypothyroidism. Because it increases metabolic rate, it should be taken in the morning to minimise the occurrence of insomnia. Common side-effects of metformin are gastrointestinal, such as nausea and vomiting. By taking the tablet with or after food, these side-effects are minimised. Dipyridamole should be taken three times daily before food, as dipyridamole is incompletely absorbed from the gastrointestinal tract.

A76   D

Hypothyroidism occurs in the older population and may have an insidious onset. Signs and symptoms of hypothyroidism tend to be subacute and presentation may be related to non-specific symptoms.

A77   D

When thyroxine is administered to patients receiving warfarin, it enhances the anticoagulant effect of warfarin.

A78   A

Caution should be undertaken when thyroxine is started in elderly patients and in patients with cardiovascular disorders, as there could be a rapid increase in metabolic rate leading to problems including anginal pain, arrhythmias, palpitations, tachycardia. In diabetic patients, caution should be used, as its introduction may interfere with antidiabetic therapy. It should be started in small doses at small increments.

A79   B

Side-effects resemble symptoms of hyperthyroidism and include diarrhoea, anginal pain, tachycardia, skeletal muscle cramps, tremors, restlessness, excitability, insomnia, headache and flushing.

A80   D

The thyroid hormones T_3 and T_4 are transported in the blood by three proteins: the thyroid-binding globulin; thyroid-binding prealbumin; and albumin. Hence the total thyroid hormones concentration in plasma changes with alterations in amount of thyroxine-binding in plasma. Only the unbound thyroid hormone is able to diffuse into the thyroid cell and elicit a biological response. For this reason the concentration of total thyroid hormones in plasma is not considered a good diagnostic marker. Laboratory investigations to diagnose and monitor management of hypothyroidism are based on free T_3, free T_4 and thyroid-stimulating hormone (TSH). In the early stages of hypothyroidism, free T_3 and free T_4 concentrations may be normal and a modest increase in TSH is detected. Free T_3 and free T_4 may decline as the disease progresses.

Test 2

Questions

Questions 1-6

Directions: Each group of questions below consists of five lettered headings followed by a list of numbered questions. For each numbered question select the one heading that is most closely related to it. Each heading may be used once, more than once, or not at all.

Questions 1-3 concern the following abbreviations:

A   ☐ PMH
B   ☐ O/E
C   ☐ SH
D   ☐ PC
E   ☐ FH

Select, from A to E, which one of the above:

Q1   is a description of conditions that the patient has experienced previously

Q2   is symptoms presented by the patient

Q3   is the findings of examination of the patient

Questions 4-6 concern the following abbreviations:

A   ☐ HbA1c
B   ☐ BUN
C   ☐ TSH
D   ☐ LFT
E   ☐ MCV

Select, from A to E, which one of the above:

Q4   is carried out as part of kidney function monitoring

Q5   is carried out in thyroid function monitoring

Q6   is used to monitor diabetic patients

Questions 7–26

Directions: For each of the questions below, ONE or MORE of the responses is (are) correct. Decide which of the responses is (are) correct. Then choose:

A   ☐ if 1, 2 and 3 are correct
B   ☐ if 1 and 2 only are correct
C   ☐ if 2 and 3 only are correct
D   ☐ if 1 only is correct
E   ☐ if 3 only is correct

Directions summarised				
A	B	C	D	E
1, 2, 3	1, 2 only	2, 3 only	1 only	3 only

Q7   INR:

1   ☐ is monitored in patients with arthritis
2   ☐ is monitored in patients receiving warfarin
3   ☐ stands for international normalised ratio

Q8   Lung function tests:

1   ❑ always involve administration of bronchodilators before the procedure

2   ❑ are used to determine severity of respiratory disease

3   ❑ are used to monitor outcomes of therapy

Q9   In heart failure:

1   ❑ chest radiographs may show cardiac enlargement

2   ❑ the pulse rate may indicate arrhythmias

3   ❑ body extremities are very hot

Q10   Colonoscopy:

1   ❑ is an artificial opening between the colon and skin

2   ❑ should not be performed in periods of less than five years

3   ❑ requires the patient to perform bowel cleansing

Q11   EEG:

1   ❑ is carried out to confirm the occurrence of cardiovascular disease

2   ❑ procedures require patients to be totally sedated

3   ❑ stands for electroencephalography

Q12   Chronically elevated arterial pressure may cause:

1   ❑ renovascular disease

2   ❑ haemorrhagic stroke

3   ❑ nasal congestion

Q13   Atherosclerosis:

1   ❑ can occur in different organs

2   ❑ may result in myocardial infarction

3   ❑ causes chest pain

Q14 Patients with angina pectoris may be advised that factors which precipitate an attack include:

1 ☐ exercise
2 ☐ anxiety
3 ☐ light meals

Q15 After a myocardial infarction, a patient should be advised:

1 ☐ that normal activity can never be re-achieved
2 ☐ to attain normal body weight
3 ☐ to undertake moderate exercise

Q16 Common complications of gallstones include:

1 ☐ biliary colic
2 ☐ jaundice
3 ☐ appendicitis

Q17 Patients with osteoarthritis should be informed that:

1 ☐ disease progression is very gradual
2 ☐ weight loss is recommended
3 ☐ prolonged bed-rest is advisable

Q18 Patients receiving cytotoxic chemotherapy should be advised that:

1 ☐ nausea and vomiting may occur before treatment
2 ☐ hair loss may occur
3 ☐ any signs of infection should be reported to a health professional

Q19 When a patient presents with a fall and a blackout:

1 ☐ the incident has to be investigated
2 ☐ the patient has epilepsy
3 ☐ the incident should raise the alarm only if it occurs in paediatric patients

Q20   Hypokalaemia may be due to:

1   ☐ vomiting
2   ☐ drugs
3   ☐ renal failure

Q21   Clinical features of hypoglycaemia include:

1   ☐ sweating
2   ☐ hunger
3   ☐ blurred vision

Q22   An anaphylactic shock could present with:

1   ☐ rash
2   ☐ bronchoconstriction
3   ☐ hypertension

Q23   Diabetic patients should be advised to monitor their condition because they are prone to develop:

1   ☐ retinopathy
2   ☐ chronic renal failure
3   ☐ ischaemic heart disease

Q24   Normal saline:

1   ☐ is 0.9% sodium chloride
2   ☐ may be used in electrolyte imbalance
3   ☐ may be applied as nasal drops

Q25   Disadvantages of the administration of corticosteroids in the eye include:

1   ☐ corneal thinning
2   ☐ glaucoma
3   ☐ cataracts

Q26 In which of the following cases is referral recommended?

1 ☐ an asthmatic patient who presents with fever, chesty cough and wheezing

2 ☐ a patient receiving antihypertensive medication who presents with nasal congestion

3 ☐ a patient presenting with allergic rhinitis

Questions 27–80

Directions: These questions involve cases. Read the case description or patient profile and answer the questions. For questions with one or more correct answers, follow the key given with each question. For the other questions, only one answer is correct – give the corresponding answer.

Questions 27–38 involve the following case:

AB is a 74-year-old male admitted to a medical ward.

PMH diabetes mellitus controlled by diet
hypertension
congestive heart failure

DH bumetanide 1 mg daily
potassium chloride 600 mg bd
isosorbide dinitrate 10 mg tds
atenolol 100 mg bd
aspirin 75 mg daily
lorazepam 1 mg tds
metoclopramide 10 mg prn

PC increasing shortness of breath
dyspnoea, cyanosis, tachycardia

O/E BP 160/100 mmHg
pulse 100 bpm

Diagnosis   congestive heart failure
Lab   sodium 130 mmol/l (135–145)
        potassium 3.2 mmol/l (3.5–5.0)
        chloride 95 mmol/l (96–106)
        fasting blood glucose 15.6 mmol/l (3.6–6.0)

Drug treatment on discharge:
        bumetanide 1 mg daily
        isosorbide dinitrate 10 mg tds
        enalapril 5 mg nocte
        aspirin 75 mg daily
        lorazepam 1 mg tds
        metoclopramide 10 mg prn

Q27   What condition(s) does AB have?

1   ☐   asthma
2   ☐   diabetes mellitus
3   ☐   congestive heart failure

A   ☐   1, 2, 3
B   ☐   1, 2 only
C   ☐   2, 3 only
D   ☐   1 only
E   ☐   3 only

Q28   Signs and symptoms of congestive heart failure include:

1   ☐   oedema
2   ☐   dyspnoea
3   ☐   insomnia

A   ☐   1, 2, 3
B   ☐   1, 2 only
C   ☐   2, 3 only
D   ☐   1 only
E   ☐   3 only

Q29   Bumetanide is a (an):

A   ☐ thiazide diuretic
B   ☐ loop diuretic
C   ☐ potassium-sparing diuretic
D   ☐ aldosterone antagonist
E   ☐ osmotic diuretic

Q30   Isosorbide dinitrate:

1   ☐ is used for prophylaxis of angina
2   ☐ is metabolised to isosorbide mononitrate
3   ☐ can only be administered sublingually

A   ☐ 1, 2, 3
B   ☐ 1, 2 only
C   ☐ 2, 3 only
D   ☐ 1 only
E   ☐ 3 only

Q31   Atenolol:

1   ☐ is a beta-adrenoceptor blocking drug
2   ☐ is contraindicated in uncontrolled heart failure
3   ☐ maximum daily dose is 100 mg

A   ☐ 1, 2, 3
B   ☐ 1, 2 only
C   ☐ 2, 3 only
D   ☐ 1 only
E   ☐ 3 only

Q32   Lorazepam:

1   ☐ has a sedative effect
2   ☐ is used to alleviate anxiety
3   ☐ may cause ataxia in AB

A   ☐ 1, 2, 3
B   ☐ 1, 2 only
C   ☐ 2, 3 only
D   ☐ 1 only
E   ☐ 3 only

Q33   AB was started on enalapril because it:

1   ☐ has a valuable role in heart failure
2   ☐ lowers blood pressure
3   ☐ prevents myocardial infarction

A   ☐ 1, 2, 3
B   ☐ 1, 2 only
C   ☐ 2, 3 only
D   ☐ 1 only
E   ☐ 3 only

Q34   When starting AB on enalapril, the following parameters should be monitored:

1   ☐ blood pressure
2   ☐ serum potassium levels
3   ☐ kidney function

A   ☐ 1, 2, 3
B   ☐ 1, 2 only
C   ☐ 2, 3 only
D   ☐ 1 only
E   ☐ 3 only

Q35   Upon discharge patient is informed that:

1   ☐ his medication has been reviewed
2   ☐ instead of atenolol he is prescribed enalapril to be taken
         daily at night
3   ☐ he should take metoclopramide only as required

A   ☐ 1, 2, 3
B   ☐ 1, 2 only
C   ☐ 2, 3 only
D   ☐ 1 only
E   ☐ 3 only

Q36   Regarding bumetanide, AB should be advised to take:

1   ☐ one tablet daily
2   ☐ dose in the morning
3   ☐ dose on an empty stomach

A   ☐ 1, 2, 3
B   ☐ 1, 2 only
C   ☐ 2, 3 only
D   ☐ 1 only
E   ☐ 3 only

Q37   The patient should be advised to take isosorbide dinitrate tablets at:

A   ☐ 8 am, 2 pm, 6 pm
B   ☐ 8 am, 4 pm, 1 am
C   ☐ 8 am, 3 pm, 10 pm
D   ☐ 7 am, 3 pm, 2 am
E   ☐ 7 am, 3 pm, midnight

Q38   Follow-up of AB includes monitoring of:

1   ❑ blood pressure
2   ❑ blood glucose levels
3   ❑ development of oedema

A   ❑ 1, 2, 3
B   ❑ 1, 2 only
C   ❑ 2, 3 only
D   ❑ 1 only
E   ❑ 3 only

Questions 39–40 involve the following case:

XY is a 49-year-old patient who is allergic to penicillin. She was prescribed erythromycin for cellulitis. She developed a rash and erythromycin was withdrawn.

Q39   Which of the following antibacterial agents is the most appropriate for XY:

A   ❑ flucloxacillin
B   ❑ cefuroxime
C   ❑ nalidixic acid
D   ❑ fluconazole
E   ❑ isoniazid

Q40   When XY is started on the new treatment:

1   ❑ development of a rash should be monitored
2   ❑ signs of anaphylaxis should be detected
3   ❑ an allergic reaction could develop after a month after last drug administration

A ☐ 1, 2, 3
B ☐ 1, 2 only
C ☐ 2, 3 only
D ☐ 1 only
E ☐ 3 only

Questions 41–42 involve the following case:

PS is a 69-year-old patient who presents with orofacial unwanted movements. His
medication includes diazepam 5 mg nocte and amitriptyline 25 mg tds

Q41   The presenting complaint could be:

A ☐ akathisia
B ☐ tardive dyskinesia
C ☐ agranulocytosis
D ☐ purpura
E ☐ hypomania

Q42   A review of medication could propose changing amitriptyline to:

1 ☐ imipramine
2 ☐ venlafaxine
3 ☐ reboxetine

A ☐ 1, 2, 3
B ☐ 1, 2 only
C ☐ 2, 3 only
D ☐ 1 only
E ☐ 3 only

Questions 43–47 involve the following case:

QR is a 75-year-old male whose current medication is:
  co-codamol 2 tablets qid
  paracetamol 1 g qid
  gliclazide 80 mg bd
  ferrous sulphate 800 mg tds
  dipyridamole 25 mg tds
  isosorbide dinitrate 20 mg tds

Q43   Pharmacist intervention includes:

1   ❏   suggesting cessation of co-codamol
2   ❏   reviewing the dose of ferrous sulphate
3   ❏   reviewing the isosorbide dinitrate dose as the maximum
            daily dose is 5 mg daily

A   ❏   1, 2, 3
B   ❏   1, 2 only
C   ❏   2, 3 only
D   ❏   1 only
E   ❏   3 only

Q44   The maximum adult daily dose of paracetamol is:

A   ❏   1 g
B   ❏   2 g
C   ❏   3 g
D   ❏   4 g
E   ❏   8 g

Q45   Gliclazide:

A   ☐   augments insulin secretion
B   ☐   can only be used as monotherapy
C   ☐   promotes weight loss
D   ☐   causes hyperglycaemia
E   ☐   inhibits intestinal alpha-glucosidases

Q46   The patient should be advised:

1   ☐   to take small, frequent meals
2   ☐   to avoid a high-calorie diet
3   ☐   to consume food with a high fat content

A   ☐   1, 2, 3
B   ☐   1, 2 only
C   ☐   2, 3 only
D   ☐   1 only
E   ☐   3 only

Q47   QR is receiving medication to achieve:

1   ☐   analgesia
2   ☐   an antiplatelet effect
3   ☐   coronary vasodilation

A   ☐   1, 2, 3
B   ☐   1, 2 only
C   ☐   2, 3 only
D   ☐   1 only
E   ☐   3 only

Questions 48–51 involve the following case:

MR is an 82-year-old female hospitalised at the ophthalmic ward. Her current medication is:
   framycetin eye drops 1 drop both eyes tds
   dorzolamide eye drops 1 drop left eye bd
   acetazolamide tablets 125 mg bd
   timolol eye drops 0.5% 1 drop left eye bd
   ranitidine tablets 150 mg nocte
   bisacodyl tablets 5 mg daily

Q48   Use of bisacodyl in MR requires assessment because it can:

1   ❏ precipitate atonic colon
2   ❏ precipitate hypokalaemia
3   ❏ cause intestinal obstruction

A   ❏ 1, 2, 3
B   ❏ 1, 2 only
C   ❏ 2, 3 only
D   ❏ 1 only
E   ❏ 3 only

Q49   In MR bisacodyl could be replaced with:

A   ❏ senna
B   ❏ docusate sodium
C   ❏ liquid paraffin
D   ❏ magnesium hydroxide
E   ❏ lactulose

Q50   Framycetin drug therapy:

1   ☐   is used to treat eye infection
2   ☐   may be used for prophylaxis following eye surgery
3   ☐   is used short-term

A   ☐   1, 2, 3
B   ☐   1, 2 only
C   ☐   2, 3 only
D   ☐   1 only
E   ☐   3 only

Q51   Condition(s) being treated in the left eye only:

1   ☐   cataract
2   ☐   infection
3   ☐   glaucoma

A   ☐   1, 2, 3
B   ☐   1, 2 only
C   ☐   2, 3 only
D   ☐   1 only
E   ☐   3 only

Questions 52–53 involve the following case:

CB, a 59-year-old male was admitted to hospital with a severe chest infection. His current medication is

lactulose 30 ml daily

warfarin 4 mg daily adjusted according to INR

paracetamol 500 mg prn

CB is allergic to penicillin and suffers from tinnitus and hearing loss.

Q52   Which of the following antibacterial preparations is the most appropriate?

A   ☐   co-amoxiclav
B   ☐   cefuroxime
C   ☐   gentamicin
D   ☐   ciprofloxacin
E   ☐   sodium fusidate

Q53   Lactulose:

1   ☐   treatment in CB should be withdrawn
2   ☐   is used for chronic constipation
3   ☐   may cause flatulence

A   ☐   1, 2, 3
B   ☐   1, 2 only
C   ☐   2, 3 only
D   ☐   1 only
E   ☐   3 only

Questions 54–58 involve the following case:

JM is a 40-year-old female in the terminal stages of carcinoma. Her current medication is:
    paroxetine 20 mg daily
    tamoxifen 20 mg daily
    co-codamol 2 tabs tds
    diazepam 2 mg nocte
JM is still complaining of pain.

Q54   Which of the following is an alternative treatment to co-codamol?

A   ❑ domperidone
B   ❑ paracetamol
C   ❑ morphine
D   ❑ aspirin
E   ❑ ibuprofen

Q55   What side-effects could be expected from analgesics used for palliative care?

1   ❑ nausea
2   ❑ vomiting
3   ❑ constipation

A   ❑ 1, 2, 3
B   ❑ 1, 2 only
C   ❑ 2, 3 only
D   ❑ 1 only
E   ❑ 3 only

Q56   Tamoxifen:

1   ❑ is used in breast cancer
2   ❑ is associated with the occurrence of hot flushes
3   ❑ is administered every 2 weeks

A   ❑ 1, 2, 3
B   ❑ 1, 2 only
C   ❑ 2, 3 only
D   ❑ 1 only
E   ❑ 3 only

Q57   Paroxetine:

1   ☐   is used in JM to alleviate depression and anxiety
2   ☐   dose is given in the morning
3   ☐   is administered with or after food

A   ☐   1, 2, 3
B   ☐   1, 2 only
C   ☐   2, 3 only
D   ☐   1 only
E   ☐   3 only

Q58   In JM the disadvantages of diazepam are:

1   ☐   withdrawal symptoms
2   ☐   dependence
3   ☐   confusion

A   ☐   1, 2, 3
B   ☐   1, 2 only
C   ☐   2, 3 only
D   ☐   1 only
E   ☐   3 only

Questions 59–60 involve the following case:

LX is an 82-year-old female who is admitted with an infection in the right toe. On admission her medication is:

dipyridamole 100 mg tds
aspirin 75 mg daily
glibenclamide 5 mg bd

Her fasting blood glucose level was 12 mmol/l (3.6–6.0 mmol/l). LX was started on:

 cefuroxime 750 mg iv 8 hourly
 metronidazole 500 mg iv 8 hourly
 insulin according to blood glucose levels

Glibenclamide was stopped.

Q59   Reasons for the change in antidiabetic therapy:

1   ☐   diabetes is not controlled
2   ☐   to remove oral drug administration
3   ☐   LX has stopped intake of food

A   ☐   1, 2, 3
B   ☐   1, 2 only
C   ☐   2, 3 only
D   ☐   1 only
E   ☐   3 only

Q60   Metronidazole was included in the therapeutic regimen:

1   ☐   to cover against anaerobic bacteria
2   ☐   to potentiate cefuroxime
3   ☐   for a topical effect

A   ☐   1, 2, 3
B   ☐   1, 2 only
C   ☐   2, 3 only
D   ☐   1 only
E   ☐   3 only

Questions 61–62 involve the following case:

FS has been prescribed 50 mg morphine sulphate in the morning and 100 mg morphine sulphate at night. The preferred route of administration for FS is oral tablets and morphine sulphate is available as tablets of 10 mg, 30 mg, and 60 mg.

Q61 How many morphine sulphate tablets need to be dispensed for a morning dose?

1 ☐ one 30 mg tablet
2 ☐ two 10 mg tablets
3 ☐ three 10 mg tablets

A ☐ 1, 2, 3
B ☐ 1, 2 only
C ☐ 2, 3 only
D ☐ 1 only
E ☐ 3 only

Q62 How many morphine sulphate tablets need to be dispensed for the evening dose?

1 ☐ one 60 mg tablet
2 ☐ one 10 mg tablet
3 ☐ one 30 mg tablet

A ☐ 1, 2, 3
B ☐ 1, 2 only
C ☐ 2, 3 only
D ☐ 1 only
E ☐ 3 only

Questions 63–65 involve the following case:

CP is a 28-year-old male who presents with complaints of weakness, dizziness and sweating. CP had undergone a gastroscopy, which revealed a duodenal ulcer. He tested negative to the *Helicobacter pylori* urea breath test. Laboratory tests confirm that CP is found to have anaemia. His medication on admission is
   gliclazide 40 mg daily
   esomeprazole 20 mg daily
   aluminium–magnesium containing antacid 10 ml qid

Q63   A likely cause of anaemia in CP is:

A   ☐ gastrointestinal haemorrhage
B   ☐ splenomegaly
C   ☐ inadequate diet
D   ☐ autoimmune disease
E   ☐ congenital disease

Q64   Actions to be taken for CP include:

1   ☐ start ferrous sulphate tablets
2   ☐ administer iron sorbitol injection
3   ☐ carry out gastric lavage

A   ☐ 1, 2, 3
B   ☐ 1, 2 only
C   ☐ 2, 3 only
D   ☐ 1 only
E   ☐ 3 only

Q65   On discharge CP should be advised:

1   ☐ to avoid NSAIDs
2   ☐ to take small frequent meals
3   ☐ to reduce intake of fibre

A ☐ 1, 2, 3
B ☐ 1, 2 only
C ☐ 2, 3 only
D ☐ 1 only
E ☐ 3 only

Questions 66–72 involve the following case:

MC is an 84-year-old female referred to the A&E department with gradual deterioration in her general condition. Patient is not eating or drinking for the past few days.

PMH	diabetes mellitus, congestive heart failure, ischaemic heart disease, dementia
DH	perindopril 2 mg daily
	digoxin 0.0625 mg daily
	bumetanide 1 mg daily
	metformin 500 mg bd
	amitriptyline 20 mg nocte
	ranitidine 150 mg daily
SH	lives alone, ° smoking, ° alcohol
O/E	° SOB, ° sputum, ° cough
	pressure sore over sacrum and heels
	BP: 170/110 mmHg
	pulse: 120 bpm
	sparse bilateral inspiratory crackles
	poor respiratory effort
	abdomen soft non tender
	° oedema
LaB	WBC 8 × 10⁹/l (5–10 × 10⁹/l)
Impression	dehydrated ++, early parkinsonian features

Patient is started on intravenous 0.9% saline 1 litre, alternating with 5% dextrose 1 litre 8 hourly at the A&E department and admitted to hospital.

Q66   Features that could have caused the onset of dehydration in MC:

1   ❑ amitriptyline
2   ❑ bumetanide
3   ❑ low fluid intake

A   ❑ 1, 2, 3
B   ❑ 1, 2 only
C   ❑ 2, 3 only
D   ❑ 1 only
E   ❑ 3 only

Q67   The poor health, poor respiratory effort and bilateral inspiratory crackles suggest the need to start:

1   ❑ prednisolone iv
2   ❑ budesonide by inhalation
3   ❑ co-amoxiclav iv

A   ❑ 1, 2, 3
B   ❑ 1, 2 only
C   ❑ 2, 3 only
D   ❑ 1 only
E   ❑ 3 only

Q68   What measures need to be undertaken during parenteral rehydration?

1   ❑ monitor blood sodium levels
2   ❑ monitor blood glucose 6 hourly
3   ❑ stop bumetanide

A   ❑ 1, 2, 3
B   ❑ 1, 2 only
C   ❑ 2, 3 only
D   ❑ 1 only
E   ❑ 3 only

Q69   With regards to the use of metformin, MC should be advised:

1   ☐   to take tablets with meals
2   ☐   to avoid alcoholic drink
3   ☐   that soft stools occur usually as a long-term side-effect

A   ☐   1, 2, 3
B   ☐   1, 2 only
C   ☐   2, 3 only
D   ☐   1 only
E   ☐   3 only

Q70   Amitriptyline:

1   ☐   is more sedative than imipramine
2   ☐   a reduced dose is recommended for older persons
3   ☐   its use in MC should be revised because of her medical history

A   ☐   1, 2, 3
B   ☐   1, 2 only
C   ☐   2, 3 only
D   ☐   1 only
E   ☐   3 only

Q71   Early parkinsonian features include:

1   ☐   bradykinesia
2   ☐   incontinence
3   ☐   postural instability

A   ☐   1, 2, 3
B   ☐   1, 2 only
C   ☐   2, 3 only
D   ☐   1 only
E   ☐   3 only

Q72   In MC:

1   ❑ parkinsonian symptoms may be precipitated by amitriptyline
2   ❑ physiotherapy may provide patient support to counteract onset of parkinsonian symptoms
3   ❑ signs of dementia exclude occurrence of Parkinson's disease

A   ❑ 1, 2, 3
B   ❑ 1, 2 only
C   ❑ 2, 3 only
D   ❑ 1 only
E   ❑ 3 only

Questions 73–75 involve the following case:

BC is a 9-year-old female who has been on holiday at a seaside resort for a week. She presents with her parents and is complaining of a red, scaly skin area on both her elbows. The area has a golden-yellow crust and BC complains that it is very itchy. BC suffers from atopic eczema.

Q73   Possibilities of diagnosis include:

1   ❑ exacerbation of atopic eczema
2   ❑ impetigo
3   ❑ ringworm infection

A   ❑ 1, 2, 3
B   ❑ 1, 2 only
C   ❑ 2, 3 only
D   ❑ 1 only
E   ❑ 3 only

Q74 Drugs that could be recommended for use in BC include:

1 ☐ hydrocortisone 1% cream
2 ☐ mepyramine cream
3 ☐ miconazole cream

A ☐ 1, 2, 3
B ☐ 1, 2 only
C ☐ 2, 3 only
D ☐ 1 only
E ☐ 3 only

Q75 The parents of BC should be reminded to:

1 ☐ avoid use of soaps and bubble baths
2 ☐ use hypoallergenic sun protection cream
3 ☐ ensure good hydration

A ☐ 1, 2, 3
B ☐ 1, 2 only
C ☐ 2, 3 only
D ☐ 1 only
E ☐ 3 only

Questions 76–80 involve the following case:

GM is a 28-year-old female who suffers from tension headache. She would like to have a medication that is stronger than paracetamol.

Q76 Tension headache:

1 ☐ tends to have a chronic pattern
2 ☐ is due to arterial vasoconstriction
3 ☐ occurs only in young adults

A ☐ 1, 2, 3
B ☐ 1, 2 only
C ☐ 2, 3 only
D ☐ 1 only
E ☐ 3 only

Q77   Characteristic complaints of patients with tension headache are:

1 ☐ feeling of a bilateral 'hatband'
2 ☐ pain is non-throbbing
3 ☐ sound intolerance

A ☐ 1, 2, 3
B ☐ 1, 2 only
C ☐ 2, 3 only
D ☐ 1 only
E ☐ 3 only

Q78   GM could be advised to:

1 ☐ adopt a less stressful life
2 ☐ avoid consumption of cheese
3 ☐ change employment

A ☐ 1, 2, 3
B ☐ 1, 2 only
C ☐ 2, 3 only
D ☐ 1 only
E ☐ 3 only

Q79   Analgesics that could be recommended to GM include:

1 ☐ co-codamol
2 ☐ ibuprofen
3 ☐ amitriptyline

A ❏ 1, 2, 3
B ❏ 1, 2 only
C ❏ 2, 3 only
D ❏ 1 only
E ❏ 3 only

Q80   The use of aspirin would not be recommended if GM:

1 ❏ has hypertension
2 ❏ has a history of gastric ulceration
3 ❏ is breast-feeding

A ❏ 1, 2, 3
B ❏ 1, 2 only
C ❏ 2, 3 only
D ❏ 1 only
E ❏ 3 only

Test 2

Answers

Questions 1–3

Abbreviations are commonly encountered in case notes. They are standardised to help exchange of information between different health care settings and so that case notes can be used by different health professionals.

A1　A

PMH stands for *past medical history*, where information on conditions experienced previously by the patient is reported.

A2　D

PC stands for *presenting complaint*, where the symptoms that are reported by the patient are included.

A3　B

O/E stands for *on examination*, where the information observed by health professionals is noted.

Questions 4–6

Clinical laboratory tests are significant in chronic disease management to monitor outcomes of therapy and compliance with pharmacotherapy and lifestyle measures.

A4   B

BUN stands for *blood urea nitrogen*. It provides an indirect measure of renal function and glomerular filtration rate, and also gauges liver function. Urea is formed in the liver as an end-product of protein metabolism. Urea is transported to the kidneys for excretion. For kidney function monitoring it should not be used as a stand-alone test, because changes in the metabolic function of the liver could affect the BUN results. BUN is used together with creatinine levels in the monitoring of kidney function.

A5   C

TSH stands for *thyroid-stimulating hormone*, and its concentrations are monitored in thyroid disease.

A6   A

HbA1c, also referred to as glycosylated haemoglobin, is used to monitor diabetes. It measures the blood glucose bound to haemoglobin. As erythrocytes have a life span of 120 days, the test reflects the average blood sugar level in the 2–3 months preceding the test. It gives an indication of the blood glucose levels over the past 90 days.

Questions 7–26

A7   C

INR stands for *international normalised ratio*. It is a ratio value comparing a patient's prothrombin time against the prothrombin time of normal control patients. It is used as a monitoring index in patients receiving warfarin. INR levels for patients on warfarin are aimed at between two and three, depending on the goal of treatment and other factors, such as recurrent deep vein thrombosis or use of prosthetic heart valves.

A8   C

Lung function tests involve the use of a spirometer to measure lung volumes and air flow rates. Measurements include forced expiratory volume, vital capacity, forced vital capacity and residual volume. Lung function tests are used to determine the severity of the respiratory disease and to monitor outcomes of therapy. Patients may be educated to use a patient-friendly spirometer device to monitor their condition and adjust their therapy accordingly as advised by the healthcare team. Lung function tests may be used to determine the reversibility of airway disease. Sometimes a bronchodilator may be administered before the procedure after baseline pulmonary function tests have been carried out, to evaluate the degree of disease reversibility.

A9   B

Heart failure results in a reduced cardiac output leading to impaired oxygenation and a compromised blood supply to muscles. A common cause of heart failure is left ventricular systolic dysfunction. Sustained heart failure results in compensatory mechanisms by the body to maintain circulation. These result in long-term sequelae such as remodelling of the left ventricle and cardiac enlargement. A chest radiograph may reveal an enlarged cardiac shadow and consolidation in the lungs. Due to the occurrence of cardiomegaly, arrhythmias may occur. Patients with heart failure present with dyspnoea or orthopnoea, may appear pale and may have cold extremities.

A10   E

Colonoscopy is a diagnostic procedure that is used in the assessment of gastrointestinal disorders of the colon. It may be used to diagnose inflammatory bowel disease and carcinoma. It is used to assess the management of patients with inflammatory bowel disease; for example, in patients who have undergone surgery for ulcerative colitis, regular colonoscopy is undertaken to evaluate recurrence of the disease. It is also used as a diagnostic screening tool in familial colon cancer. It may be repeated as necessary. A disadvantage is that bowel cleansing is required before the procedure and if this is not done efficiently then the results are compromised.

A11   E

EEG stands for *electroencephalography* and it is a test carried out to measure and record electrical impulses in the brain. It is used to diagnose seizures. However the EEG has limitations and patients with epilepsy may present with a normal EEG, but the EEG helps in classifying seizures. The procedure may be carried out in a sleep-induced state or in a sleep-deprived state.

A12   B

Arterial pressure reflects the stress exerted by the circulating blood on the arterial walls. It is directly related to the cardiac output and the systemic vascular resistance. In chronically elevated arterial blood pressure, direct organ and vascular damage may result, caused by increased peripheral resistance and by arteriosclerosis. Organs commonly affected include the heart, kidneys, brain and retina. Manifestations of the sustained damage are renovascular disease, such as renal failure; cerebrovascular disease, such as thrombotic stroke; retinal damage resulting in visual defects; and cardio-vascular disease, such as ischaemic heart disease.

A13   B

Atherosclerosis is a common arterial disorder characterised by deposits of plaques consisting of cholesterol, lipids and cellular debris on the inner layers of walls of large- and medium-sized arteries. It may occur in any artery and increases the risk of thrombosis. It is a cause of coronary artery disease, angina and myocardial infarction. Its occurrence increases with age and is related to smoking, obesity, hypertension, diabetes mellitus and elevated low-density lipoprotein cholesterol levels.

A14   B

Angina pectoris is thoracic pain, most often caused by myocardial anoxia. Symptoms of angina pectoris may occur with activities or circumstances that increase cardiac workload such as: exertion following exercise, like climbing stairs; emotion, such as anxiety, which results in an increased heart rate; heavy meals, because of the requirement of increased gastrointestinal perfusion; and exposure to cold temperatures owing to peripheral vasoconstriction, which leads to increased peripheral resistance.

A15   C

A myocardial infarction occurs because of a coronary vessel occlusion for a duration of about 6 h. Infarct size may be limited by dilatation of neighbouring vessels brought about by a mechanism of autoregulation. Myocardial infarction is caused by atherosclerosis and the patient presents with severe, crushing, retrosternal pain. In the absence of complications, patients resume mobilisation within 2 or 3 days of a myocardial infarction. Subsequently patients should be advised to follow a healthy diet which is low in fats, to undertake routine exercise and to attain a normal body weight. They should be reassured that a gradual re-establishment of normal activity will be achieved. Family and friends should be counselled how to help the patient achieve this.

A16   B

Gallstones consist of cholesterol and bile pigments that are calcified. Common complications of gallstones include biliary colic, cholestatic jaundice, acute pancreatitis and acute cholecystitis and cholangitis. In biliary colic the patient complains of moderate to severe pain in the epigastric area. Jaundice occurs because of obstruction of the bile ducts and presents with generalised pruritus. In acute pancreatitis there is reflux of the bile up the pancreatic duct and it causes pain and vomiting. Acute cholecystitis and cholangitis are due to inflammation of the gall bladder and common bile duct.

A17   B

In osteoarthritis degenerative changes including subchondral bony sclerosis, loss of articular cartilage and proliferation of bone spurs occur in one or many joints. As the disease progresses inflammation of the synovial membrane takes place. The disease is not reversible except where joint replacement is undertaken. However, disease progression is very gradual and patients should be advised how to rest and support involved joints through proper physiotherapist-guided exercises. Losing weight helps to reduce stress on the joints.

A18   C

A major disadvantage of cytotoxic chemotherapy is that it interferes with cellular activity in cancerous and normal tissues. It is associated with unwanted effects because of its effect on normal cells. Nausea and vomiting after treatment are very common side-effects. Their extent depends on the emetogenic potential of the drugs used. When these side-effects are not very well controlled, there is a risk that the patient develops anticipatory nausea and vomiting before treatment. However, this effect is psychologically and not chemically induced. Alopecia, which is usually reversible, is another common side-effect. Because of the suppressive effects on the bone-marrow caused by cytotoxic chemotherapy, patients are prone to develop infections. Patients should be advised to report any signs of an infection, such as sore throat or fever, to a health professional.

A19   D

When there is temporary loss of consciousness leading to a fall, it may indicate a brief cerebral hypoxia, which could be caused by a number of factors including emotional stress, vascular pooling in the legs, diaphoresis or a sudden change in body position. Such an incident may also indicate serious disease states, such as brain tumours. The patient should be assessed and medical and drug histories should be reviewed.

A20   B

Hypokalaemia is a decreased serum potassium level. Normally the potassium loss from the body through renal and faecal excretion and from loss in sweat is miminal. Hypokalaemia may result because of a high loss from the gastro-intestinal tract, as gastrointestinal secretions contain high levels of potassium. Vomiting, diarrhoea and laxative abuse could result in hypokalaemia. An increased renal clearance due to drugs, alkalosis and aldosteronism may also result in hypokalaemia. Drugs that could induce hypokalaemia include thiazide and loop diuretics and steroids. Hyperkalaemia is the excess of potassium in serum. It is commonly caused by renal failure.

A21   A

Hypoglycaemia is a blood glucose level below 3 mmol/l. It is a condition that develops rapidly and usually occurs in diabetics either because of an excessive antidiabetic dose or owing to changes in lifestyle. Patients should be educated to identify symptoms of hypoglycaemia so that they can counteract it by taking carbohydrates, to prevent neuroglycopenic symptoms such as drowsiness, disorientation and confusion progressing to convulsions, coma and death. Symptoms of hypoglycaemia indicating an activated sympathetic nervous system are sweating, tremor, pallor and anxiety. Other effects are hunger, blurred vision, salivation and weakness.

A22   B

An anaphylactic shock occurs because of a hypersensitivity reaction. Presentation includes development of a rash, acute bronchoconstriction, profound hypotension and collapse.

A23   A

Diabetes is associated with microvascular complications, the incidence of which may be reduced with optimal blood glucose control. It may lead to microvascular damage in the retina causing dilatation, haemorrhage and infarction leading to retinopathy. Retinopathy is managed with laser photo-coagulation. Its occurrence is usually associated with diabetic nephropathy. Nephropathy occurs because of sclerosis of the glomerular basement membrane. Initial signs of nephropathy are microalbuminuria, proteinuria and hypertension. ACE inhibitors are used in diabetic patients to treat hypertension as well as to dilate intrarenal vessels and thus minimise glomerular hyper-tension. Macroangiopathy occurs in cardiac vessels leading to onset of ischaemic heart disease. To decrease the effects of macroangiopathy, lipid-lowering drugs such as statins are considered in diabetic patients.

A24   A

Normal saline consists of 0.9% sodium chloride as an isotonic solution. It is used as a parenteral preparation in electrolyte and fluid imbalance such as sodium depletion. It is also available as nasal drops in nasal congestion and as a nebuliser diluent. It may be used in eye and wound irrigation and for oral hygiene.

A25   A

Topical administration of corticosteroids in the eye is associated with thinning of the cornea and sclera, steroid glaucoma and steroid cataract. These side-effects occur particularly after prolonged use. The use of a topical preparation containing only a corticosteroid in a patient presenting with a red eye may lead to aggravation of the underlying infection resulting in corneal ulceration with a possible loss of vision.

A26   D

Asthmatic patients who present with fever, chesty cough and wheezing indicate onset of a chest infection where the use of antibacterials may be necessary to counteract bacterial infections or to cover against the development of secondary bacterial infections. Referral of the patients is recommended. Patients on antihypertensive agents complaining of nasal congestion may be recommended a topical sympathomimetic drug such as xylometazoline, which will act as a vasoconstrictor and reduce the congestion with minimal systemic effects. Patients presenting with allergic rhinitis could be recommended use of systemic non-sedating antihistamine drugs such as loratidine.

Questions 27–38

AB is an elderly male patient with congestive heart failure, hypertension and diabetes. On admission he is taking bumetanide (a loop diuretic), potassium chloride, isosorbide dinitrate (a nitrate), atenolol (a beta-adrenoceptor drug), aspirin (an antiplatelet), lorazepam (an anti-anxiety drug) and metoclopramide (an anti-emetic). Potassium chloride, isosorbide dinitrate and bumetanide may cause nausea, though it is not a common side-effect. This may be the rationale behind the use of metoclopramide at night. On admission he presents with symptoms of deterioration of congestive heart failure, a high blood pressure and an elevated fasting blood glucose level.

A27   C

AB has diabetes mellitus and congestive heart failure. In elderly and diabetic patients it is very common to find multiple disease states. Metabolic stress such as deterioration of congestive heart failure may precipitate an acute disturbance in diabetic control. In AB even though there is an elevated fasting blood glucose level, this should be monitored but no therapeutic action should be taken until his cardiac condition is stabilised.

A28   B

In congestive heart failure there is generalised oedema and usually the term implies bilateral failure resulting in reduced cardiac contractility. Symptoms include oedema, dyspnoea (sensation of uncomfortable breathing) and fatigue.

A29   B

Bumetanide is a loop diuretic, which acts by inhibiting re-absorption from the ascending limb of the loop of Henle in the renal tubule. It has an onset of action within 1 h of oral administration and a duration of action of about 6 h. With regular use the impact on frequency of diuresis after drug administration tends to decrease. One of the side-effects of bumetanide is the development of hypokalaemia. Potassium supplements are administered to counteract this unwanted effect. Loop diuretics are used in the management of heart failure as they provide a symptomatic relief from the oedema. They reduce circulating blood volume and therefore decrease preload and afterload in the heart. They do not have an impact on disease progression. Had oedema been severe in AB on admission, changing bumetanide to an intravenous administration for a few days until oedema is decreased could have been an option.

A30   B

Isosorbide dinitrate is a nitrate that is used in the prophylaxis and treatment of angina and in left ventricular failure. In AB isosorbide dinitrate is being used for the management of heart failure. Nitrates cause vasodilatation and lead to a decrease in preload. Isosorbide dinitrate is metabolised to active metabolites, the most important of which is isosorbide mononitrate. It is available as short-acting tablets which may also be used sublingually in angina, as an aerosol spray, as modified-release oral dosage forms and as injection for intravenous infusion. The dose for isosorbide dinitrate in heart failure is 30–160 mg in divided doses but the dose may be increased to 240 mg daily.

A31   A

Atenolol is a cardioselective beta-adrenoceptor blocker that is used in hypertension and in angina. The recommended daily dose for atenolol in hypertension is 25–100 mg, although the 50 mg dose is usually adequate. As a beta-blocker it may mask symptoms of hypoglycaemia. However, this is of no concern in AB as the patient is not taking any antidiabetic agents but is controlling diabetes through diet. Beta-blockers have negative inotropic properties and therefore may cause bradycardia and they should not be used in patients with uncontrolled heart failure. Treatment with beta-blockers such as atenolol should be started with care in patients with heart failure. It has been demonstrated that three beta-blockers namely bisoprolol, carvedilol, and metoprolol reduce heart failure disease progression, decrease symptoms and mortality when used in stable heart failure. In AB it is an option to consider changing atenolol to an alternative therapeutic approach which better tackles the concomitant occurrence of hypertension and congestive heart failure. Use of one of these three beta-blockers (bisoprolol, carvedilol, and metoprolol) is an option.

A32   A

Lorazepam is a short-acting benzodiazepine that has anti-anxiety and hypnotic properties. Use of benzodiazepines in older people is associated with alterations in the pharmacokinetic parameters of the drug that lead to clinical consequences such as drowsiness, confusion and ataxia (a condition characterised by an inability to coordinate movement). The probability of occurrence of these side-effects is higher with drugs that have a long halflife. The use of lorazepam in AB raises concern as it appears that there is no clear rationale for its use. More data is required as to reasons for its use and duration of therapy. It may have been started recently when the patient was becoming agitated because of the insidious deterioration of his wellbeing. Owing to the onset of benzodiazepine dependence, lorazepam should not be stopped abruptly if the patient has been taking the drug for a few weeks. Abrupt withdrawal is associated with the benzodiazepine withdrawal syndrome characterised by anxiety, depression, impaired concentration, insomnia, headache and loss of appetite.

A33   B

Enalapril is an angiotensin-converting enzyme (ACE) inhibitor, which causes a decreased arterial and venous vasoconstriction and a decreased blood volume. ACE inhibitors are considered as first-line therapy in the management of heart failure because it has been shown that they reduce symptoms and improve prognosis. They are also used in hypertension as they reduce salt and water retention. The addition of enalapril to AB's therapy was an important therapeutic intervention undertaken during hospitalisation. Before admission the patient had a deterioration in the heart failure condition and required further therapeutic intervention to correct progression of the disease. By choosing to include enalapril in AB's therapy, the first-line management of congestive heart failure is now being followed.

A34   A

ACE inhibitors may cause a rapid fall in blood pressure. This may be quite relevant to AB as the patient is already being administered other drugs that have a hypotensive effect. For this reason, the first dose of ACE inhibitors should preferably be started at night so that the risk of injury caused by hypotension is lower because the patient is lying in bed. ACE inhibitors may cause hyperkalaemia and in fact the potassium chloride supplement has been stopped. ACE inhibitors may cause a deterioration in renal function, especially in patients with pre-existing disease, hypovolaemia and heart failure. When initiating treatment in AB, blood pressure, serum potassium levels and renal function should be monitored.

A35   A

Upon discharge, the changes carried out in his medications should be discussed with AB. It should be particularly pointed out that atenolol and potassium chloride have been stopped and instead enalapril has to be taken daily at night. AB should be advised to use the metoclopramide only when he has symptoms of nausea.

A36   B

Regarding bumetanide, AB should be advised to take one tablet daily in the morning to avoid waking up at night because of the increased diuresis that it causes. Bumetanide is almost completely and quite rapidly absorbed from the gastrointestinal tract and there is no need to advise patients to take the drug on an empty stomach.

A37   A

Tolerance is associated with nitrates. By reducing the nitrate concentration levels during the night, occurrence of tolerance is reduced and effectiveness maintained. Patient should receive the three doses between 7 am and 6 pm.

A38   A

Monitoring the outcome of therapy in AB is based on the measurement of blood pressure, the assessment of development of oedema and dyspnoea, and the measurement of blood glucose levels and HbA1c. A lipid profile and renal function tests could be carried out from time to time as well.

Questions 39–40

XY presents with cellulitis, which is an acute infection of the skin and sub-cutaneous tissue. It is characterised by erythema, oedema, swelling and pain and may be sometimes associated with fever, malaise and headache. Occurrence of the condition is higher where there is damaged skin, compromised circulation and in diabetics. The infection is commonly caused by Gram-positive cocci. Penicillins are the preferred antibacterial agents as first-line treatment.

A39   B

In penicillin-allergic patients, macrolides are usually the preferred drugs. Alternatively, a cephalosporin such as cefuroxime may be used with care. Some patients who are sensitive to penicillins may be also cephalosporin hypersensitive. Cephalosporins have a similar spectrum of activity to penicillins and macrolides and are usually effective against Gram-positive cocci. Cefuroxime is a second generation cephalosporin that is less susceptible to inactivation by beta-lactamases compared with first-generation cephalosporins. Flucloxacillin is a penicillinase-resistant penicillin. Nalidixic acid is a quinolone with activity predominantly against Gram-negative bacteria. Fluconazole is a triazole antifungal agent and isoniazid is an antituberculous drug. In cellulitis, when therapy is unsuccessful or inadvisable because of drug sensitivity, vancomycin may be considered.

A40   B

Hypersensitivity reactions may occur with any antibacterial agent. They are more commonly recognised with penicillins. Hypersensitivity reactions vary in presentation and may include development of a rash, an urticarial rash, fever or an acute anaphylactic reaction. Onset of allergic reaction may occur up to 14 days from first dose administration.

Questions 41–42

PS is taking diazepam, which is a benzodiazepine, and amitriptyline, which is a tricylic antidepressant. Tricyclic antidepressants may cause movement disorders and dyskinesias. There are few reports where patients using benzodiazepines developed extrapyramidal symptoms. Elderly patients may be particularly sensitive to the side-effects of benzodiazepines and tricyclic antidepressants; low doses should be used. PS is receiving the maximum dose recommended for elderly patients for amitriptyline and the lowest recommended dose for the use of diazepam in insomnia.

A41   B

PS has developed tardive dyskinesia, which is characterised by involuntary repetitive movements of muscles in the face, limbs and trunk. They may occur as a drug-induced side-effect after prolonged therapy and elderly patients are more prone to their occurrence. Withdrawal of the causative agent may result in an improvement in the condition after some time.

A42   C

Venlafaxine and reboxetine are antidepressant drugs that are less likely to be associated with the development of movement disorders. Venlafaxine is a serotonin and noradrenaline re-uptake inhibitor, whereas reboxetine is a selective inhibitor of noradrenaline. Both drugs should be used with care in patients with a history of cardiovascular disease, epilepsy, urinary retention, prostatic hypertrophy, glaucoma, renal and hepatic impairment.

Questions 43–47

QR is an elderly patient who is taking a compound preparation of codeine and paracetamol (co-codamol), paracetamol, gliclazide (sulphonylurea), ferrous sulphate, dipyridamole (antiplatelet) and isosorbide dinitrate (nitrate). A medication review is required.

A43   B

Co-codamol is a compound preparation containing paracetamol, a non-opioid analgesic, and codeine, an opioid analgesic. At the same time that he is taking this product, QR is also taking paracetamol tablets. There is overlap of therapy which could result in overdosage with paracetamol and use of codeine may lead to constipation. Pharmacist should advise QR to stop the co-codamol and continue taking only two paracetamol tablets every four hours. When normal-release ferrous sulphate tablets are used, the dose of 200 mg three times daily is recommended. For modified-release preparations, one or two tablets daily are taken. Hence the product that is being used by QR should be verified and the dose adjusted accordingly. QR could be advised to take the ferrous sulphate tablets after meals so as to decrease the occurrence of gastrointestinal irritation. QR is receiving daily 60 mg of isosorbide dinitrate, which is within the recommended dosage for isosorbide dinitrate (up to a maximum dose of 240 mg).

A44   D

The maximum adult dose of paracetamol is 4 g, administered as 0.5–1 g every 4–6 h. Overdosage with paracetamol leads to hepatic damage, which may have a delayed presentation of up to 6 days. The resulting hepatic damage may lead to encephalopathy, haemorrhage, hypoglycaemia, cerebral oedema and death. The hepatic damage is caused by a hydroxyl-ated metabolite, N-acetyl-p-benzoquinoneimine, which is usually produced in very small amounts and is detoxified by conjugation with gluthatione. In over-dosage the amount of this metabolite exceeds the gluthatione potential for detoxification.

A45   A

Gliclazide is a sulphonylurea that is used as an oral antidiabetic agent. It increases insulin secretion from functioning islet beta cells in the pancreas. Gliclazide may be used in combination with metformin (biguanide) and acarbose. Side-effects that may occur include mild gastrointestinal distur-bances such as nausea, vomiting, diarrhoea and constipation. They increase appetite and weight gain may occur. Hypoglycaemia may occur and this is relatively uncommon unless associated with overdosage or skipped meals.

A46   B

QR should be advised on healthy lifestyle measures to counteract complica-tions associated with diabetes and cardiovascular disease. These include small, frequent meals. Foods high in calories and sugar content should be avoided. QR has a higher risk of developing atherosclerosis and he should receive advice to follow a low-fat diet.

A47   A

QR is receiving analgesics (paracetamol), an antiplatelet agent (dipyridamole), and a nitrate (isosorbide dinitrate), which promote coronary vasodilation. Patient should be asked to visit health professionals regularly to have blood glucose levels, glycosylated haemoglobin, blood pressure and lipid profile assessed.

Questions 48–51

MR is receiving treatment for glaucoma with dorzolamide and acetazolamide (carbonic anhydrase inhibitors) and timolol (beta-blocker). She is receiving ranitidine, an H_2-receptor antagonist and bisacodyl which is a stimulant laxative. MR is also receiving framycetin eye drops as an antibacterial preparation.

A48   B

Bisacodyl is a diphenylmethane stimulant laxative and it acts mainly on the large intestine. Prolonged use of bisacodyl should be avoided as it may precipitate diarrhoea, hypokalaemia and atonic non-functioning colon. It may be used for the short-term management of constipation and its advantage is that it is very rapid in action. It should be avoided in intestinal obstruction and it may cause abdominal discomfort such as colic and cramps.

A49   E

In MR constipation may be a chronic problem. This is not unusual in elderly patients who have a less physically active life, may be dehydrated and may not include fibre in their diets. The problem is even more prominent if the patient is bedridden. Lactulose, which is an osmotic laxative, is a semi-synthetic disaccharide which is not absorbed from the gastrointestinal tract. It can be used in the long-term management of constipation. Senna and docusate sodium are very similar to bisacodyl. They are also stimulant laxatives. Magnesium hydroxide is not indicated for regular use. It is absorbed systemically, causes significant bowel evacuation and may cause dehydration and electrolyte imbalance. Use of liquid paraffin as a laxative is not recommended as oral administration results in anal seepage and irritation and it may give rise to foreign-body granulomatous reactions.

A50   A

Framycetin is an aminoglycoside antibacterial agent which has a bactericidal action against Gram-negative aerobic bacteria excluding *Pseudomonas* species and against some strains of staphylococci. As it is not absorbed from the gastrointestinal tract, it is used as a topical agent in skin, eye and ear infections. Usually in eye infections, topical administration of antibacterial drugs results in a positive outcome. Topical antibacterials, including framycetin, may be used for prophylaxis following ophthalmic surgical interventions. The antibacterials are used for acute management or for short-term use in prophylaxis.

A51   E

MR is receiving treatment for glaucoma, which is a raised intraocular pressure caused by obstruction of the outflow of aqueous humour. It is presented with loss of visual field. Drug therapy is aimed at decreasing intraocular pressure. Timolol, a beta-blocker, reduces intraocular pressure by reducing the rate of production of aqueous humour. Dorzolamide and acetazolamide are carbonic anhydrase inhibitors, which again interfere with the production of aqueous humour by inhibiting the enzyme involved in the process. Dorzolamide and timolol are applied topically, whereas acetazolamide is administered systemically. In glaucoma, drug therapy usually starts with monotherapy, usually either a beta-blocker or a prostaglandin analogue such as latanoprost. As the condition is monitored, combination therapy is resorted to until an optimum intraocular pressure and symptom reduction occur.

Questions 52–53

The term chest infection is usually used to refer to a lower respiratory tract infection. CB is receiving lactulose as a laxative, warfarin as an oral anti-coagulant and paracetamol as an analgesic when required. CB has ear problems with tinnitus and hearing loss.

A52   D

Ciprofloxacin is a quinolone that is active against Gram-positive and Gram-negative bacteria. It is an appropriate preparation for CB. A macrolide product such as clarithromycin is also a suitable option. As CB has a history of penicillin sensitivity, co-amoxiclav and cefuroxime should be avoided. Cefuroxime is a cephalosporin and cross-sensitivity with penicillins is possible. Gentamicin is an aminoglycoside that is not absorbed from the gastrointestinal tract and requires parenteral administration. Its use in CB is not recommended when there are other options because it may cause otoxocity as a side-effect, resulting in a deterioration in CB's ear disorders. Sodium fusidate is a narrow-spectrum product that is indicated in penicillin-resistant staphylococci infections such as osteomyelitis and in staphylococcal endocarditis.

A53   C

Lactulose is a semi-synthetic disaccharide that produces osmotic diarrhoea. It can be used for the management of chronic constipation. Its use in the acute attack is limited by the delayed onset of action (around 48 h). Side-effects of lactulose include flatulence, cramps and abdominal discomfort.

Questions 54–58

In the terminal stages of carcinoma, pain may occur because of disease progression, the debility it causes and owing to co-existing conditions. The pathophysiology of pain in terminal carcinoma may be multiple because of the varied factors leading to its occurrence. In breast cancer, bone metastases are quite common. A multidisciplinary approach should be adopted in palliative care. The pharmacist could monitor the use of drugs to maintain the patient as pain free as possible and to manage other problems such as the nausea that may arise.

A54   C

Co-codamol consists of a mixture of paracetamol, a non-opioid and codeine, an opioid drug. Codeine is effective for the relief of mild to moderate pain. An opioid drug such as morphine is required for JM. Tramadol is an opioid analgesic that is associated with fewer side-effects compared with other opioid drugs. However its use may increase risk of CNS toxicity when used together with SSRIs. Aspirin and ibuprofen are non-opioid drugs that have an anti-inflammatory and an analgesic effect. They may be of value in patients with bone pain and may be used in addition to an opioid analgesic. Domperidone is used as an anti-emetic drug. It may be required with the use of opioid drugs.

A55   A

Opioid drugs used in palliative care include tramadol and morphine. Opioids may cause nausea and vomiting especially during the initial doses, constipation and drowsiness.

A56   B

Tamoxifen is an oestrogen-receptor antagonist available as an oral formulation that is administered daily. It is used in adjuvant treatment of early breast cancer, in the palliative treatment of advanced disease and for prophylaxis in women at increased risk. The most frequent side-effect of tamoxifen is hot flushes.

A57   A

Paroxetine is a selective serotonin re-uptake inhibitor (SSRI) that is used in JM to alleviate depression and anxiety associated with terminal carcinoma. Paroxetine should be administered in the morning to minimise insomnia, anxiety and nervousness during the night. Common side-effects of SSRIs are nausea, vomiting, dyspepsia, abdominal pain, diarrhoea or constipation. Occurrence of these side-effects is reduced by administering the drug with or after food.

A58   E

Diazepam is a benzodiazepine that is associated with tolerance and dependence. The occurrence of dependence results in withdrawal symptoms, should the drug be discontinued abruptly. However, these disadvantages are not of concern in the management of JM. The aim is to keep JM pain free and in a relatively good mental state. The advantage of using diazepam as an anxiolytic outweighs the disadvantages of tolerance and dependence. A disadvantage of diazepam which is of concern in JM is the occurrence of confusion.

Questions 59–60

LX is taking dipyridamole (antiplatelet), aspirin (antiplatelet) and glibenclamide (antidiabetic agent). A complication of diabetes mellitus is vascular disease in the peripheries, which predisposes patients to the development of an infection following trauma to the area. This occurs very commonly in the feet, a condition referred to as the diabetic foot. For this reason diabetics are advised to take good care of their feet, avoid injuries and foot maceration from footwear. Diabetics should immediately seek advice about injuries to the feet to avoid development of infections in the area.

A59   D

Currently, blood glucose level is not controlled in LX. At the moment LX has an infection that is causing metabolic stress and precipitating an acute disturbance in blood glucose control. Antidiabetic treatment is changed to insulin for better control in such circumstances. Blood glucose is measured regularly for LX and insulin dose adjusted accordingly.

A60   D

Metronidazole is an anti-infective that is active against anaerobic bacteria and protozoa. It is included in the therapeutic regimen, together with cefuroxime, to expand the spectrum of activity of the anti-infectives used. Infection caused by anaerobic bacteria occurs in diabetic feet infections.

Questions 61–62

Morphine is an opioid analgesic that is widely used in the management of moderate to severe pain. It is the standard drug against which other opioid analgesics are compared. It is particularly useful in postoperative analgesia and palliative care. In addition to an analgesic effect it also induces a sense of euphoria and mental detachment. Its use may result in nausea, vomiting and constipation. Morphine may be administered as standard tablets, modified-release tablets, oral solution and injections.

A61   B

For the morning dose, FS should be given 50 mg, which can be administered as one 30 mg tablet and two 10 mg tablets. This gives the least number of tablets that the patient needs to take.

A62   A

For the evening dose, FS should be given 100 mg, which can be administered as one 60 mg tablet, one 10 mg tablet and one 30 mg tablet. This gives the least number of tablets required to be taken by the patient to achieve the required dose.

Questions 63–65

CP is receiving gliclazide (sulphonylurea), esomeprazole (proton pump inhibitor) and an antacid preparation. From this medication profile it is understood that CP is a diabetic. He has a history of duodenal ulcer disease. In the majority of cases this is caused by the organism *Helicobacter pylori* and a triple-therapy eradication regimen is recommended in these cases. However, in some patients there may be other factors that lead to duodenal ulceration. These include use of non-steroidal anti-inflammatory drugs (NSAIDs) and family history, especially when it occurs at an early age such as in the case of CP.

A63   A

In CP a cause of anaemia is gastrointestinal haemorrhage, a complication of gastric or duodenal ulcer disease, which may occur either as a minor chronic blood loss leading eventually to anaemia or as moderate bleeding leading to melaena or haematemesis. The bleeding results because of erosion of an ulcer into an artery.

A64   D

A priority in the management of CP is to correct the anaemia by administering iron supplements. Iron salts should be administered by the oral route, unless this has been unsuccessful because of non-compliance, intolerance to side-effects, malabsorption and continued blood loss. CP should be started on ferrous sulphate tablets and haemoglobin levels monitored. Iron is absorbed mostly as the ferrous state in an acidic environment and hence absorption takes place mostly in the stomach. Modified-release preparations are not recommended for CP as they do not undergo sufficient dissolution until reaching the small intestines where absorption of iron is poor. Absorption may be reduced by food; however, many patients experience nausea and diarrhoea when iron is administered on an empty stomach.

A65   B

CP should be advised to avoid non-steroidal anti-inflammatory drugs such as aspirin and to inform prescribers and pharmacists of his condition before using other medications. NSAIDs are very likely to cause gastrointestinal distress and precipitate an acute attack. He should be advised to take regular small meals, avoid strong tea, coffee and spicy food and limit food intake late at night as this increases nocturnal gastric secretion. Anxiety, stress, alcohol and smoking all contribute to precipitate duodenal ulcer disease.

Questions 66–72

MC is receiving treatment for diabetes mellitus, congestive heart failure and ischaemic heart disease. She also has a history of dementia. She is taking perindopril (angiotensin-converting enzyme inhibitor), digoxin (cardiac glycoside), bumetanide (loop diuretic), metformin (biguanide), amitriptyline (tricyclic antidepressant) and ranitidine (H_2-receptor antagonist). MC is presenting poor respiratory effort, sparse bilateral inspiratory crackles and poor general health, indicating the possibility of an underlying infection. The white blood cell count indicates that there is no leucocytosis. However, in elderly patients, bacterial infections may not necessarily induce leucocytosis.

A66   C

Onset of dehydration may be precipitated by decreased fluid intake and by loop diuretics. Risk of dehydration increases with environmental factors that support fluid and electrolyte loss, such as heat exposure caused by hot temper-atures and inadequate ventilation at home. Amitriptyline may cause dry mouth and sweating but these effects are not related to sufficient fluid loss to cause dehydration.

A67   E

In elderly patients a normal white blood cell count is not sufficient to eliminate the presence of an infection and MC has clinical signs that may indicate an infection. MC should be started on co-amoxiclav therapy intravenously. When her general condition and the respiratory features improve, treatment may be continued orally. The use of corticosteroids without the use of anti-infective agents will present a general improvement in MC but will leave the infection untreated. This is very dangerous and should be avoided.

A68   A

When MC is started on parenteral rehydration with intravenous 0.9% sodium chloride 1 litre alternating with 5% dextrose 1 litre every 8 h, blood sodium levels and blood glucose should be monitored. The bumetanide should be stopped until dehydration status is corrected, and then it should be re-introduced carefully. MC was started on sodium chloride and dextrose as she has combined electrolyte and fluid deficiency. Dextrose used alone is intended when there is fluid loss without significant loss of electrolytes. This is very uncommon.

A69   B

Metformin is an antidiabetic drug that has the advantages that it does not increase appetite and that occurrence of hypoglycaemia is very low. Its disad-vantage is that it may provoke lactic acidosis, especially in patients with renal impairment. In MC renal function should be monitored, and signs and symptoms of lactic acidosis should be noted as dehydration poses a higher risk of lactic acidosis. Side-effects of metformin include anorexia, nausea, vomiting, abdominal pain. To reduce gastrointestinal symptoms, the patient should be advised to take the drug with meals. Diarrhoea may occur initially and is only transient. When alcohol is consumed with metformin, the risk of lactic acidosis is increased. MC should be advised to avoid alcohol as it may interfere with her medications, it may precipitate dehydration and cause a deterioration in her general condition because of her dementia.

A70   A

Amitriptyline and imipramine are tricyclic antidepressants that have a tertiary amine structure. Imipramine is a dibenzazepine with a structure that is very similar to the phenothiazines, whereas amitriptyline is a dibenzocyclohepta-diene that has a structure which resembles thioxanthenes. Amitriptyline is more sedative than imipramine. Tolerance to this effect tends to develop with long-term treatment. Elderly patients may be particularly sensitive to the side-effects of tricyclic antidepressants and reduced doses are recommended. MC is taking a dose of 20 mg at night, probably to induce sleep and reduce anxiety. The dose is appropriate for the age group. Use of amitriptyline in MC requires review as its use may result in cardiotoxicity and it may alter blood-glucose concentrations, which may include hypoglycaemia unawareness. It may also cause confusion, which is a problem in MC as she also has dementia.

A71   D

MC has presented with early parkinsonian features. Bradykinesia which is general slowness of movement, is the main symptom for parkinsonism, which, during the initial phases of the disease, may occur as the only symptom or in combination with tremor at rest that disappears with activity and muscular rigidity. Postural instability is a late feature of the condition and increases the tendency to fall. As the disease progresses, patients develop reduced blink frequency, monotonous and impaired speech, greasy skin leading to sebor-rhoea, urinary incontinence and constipation.

A72 B

Amitriptyline, being a tricyclic antidepressant, may cause movement disorders and dyskinesias. Parkinsonian symptoms in MC may be precipitated by the administration of amitriptyline. The involvement of a physiotherapist in MC's healthcare team could help her to follow exercises that would delay onset of muscle rigidity and allow her to carry out normal daily activities at home with minimal support.

Questions 73–75

Eczema is a chronic inflammatory skin condition. Atopic eczema occurs mostly in children and it is characterised by pruritus, itchy papules, inflamed and lichenified skin especially on flexures such as elbows and knees. It is associated with a family history of asthma and hayfever and it may be exacerbated by allergens. The area may become infected because of pruritus, leading to a flare-up of the condition and a bacterial infection. Common causative bacteria include staphylococci and streptococci.

A73 B

BC may have an exacerbation of atopic eczema or impetigo, which is a common occurrence in patients with atopic eczema, as the area becomes infected because of the scratching that is associated with intense itching. Atopic eczema is a chronic condition that may be exacerbated by exposure to allergens such as clothing fibres, by changes in environment such as exposure to sun, hot temperatures or cold temperatures. Impetigo is a skin infection characterised by pruritic vesicles and golden-coloured crusts. It is caused by Gram-positive cocci and is a contagious condition. Ringworm infection is a fungal infection and when it occurs on non-hairy areas (tinea corporis) it is characterised by discoid, erythematous scaly plaques.

A74   D

In the management of an acute attack of atopic eczema, topical corticosteroids should be recommended. The use of 1% hydrocortisone cream is a suitable choice for BC considering that she is a child and it is a mild steroid which is rarely associated with side-effects. In addition as there is a very high probability that BC also has impetigo, a topical anti-infective agent such as fusidic acid, which is effective against Gram-positive cocci, could be administered. Topical antihistamines such as mepyramine should be avoided in eczema as they may cause hypersensitivity reactions and exacerbate the condition. Miconazole cream is an antifungal cream which is indicated for use in fungal skin infections.

A75   A

Parents of BC should be educated on the importance of preventing dehydration of the skin by ensuring good hydration and by using emollients. They should be advised on the regular use of emollients, to avoid soaps and bubble baths and to use emollient bath oils instead. They should be informed that the condition may be exacerbated by allergens such as wool, excipients in cosmetic cream preparations, and by sun exposure. They should be advised to use a hypoallergenic sun protection cream.

Questions 76–80

GM states that she suffers from tension headache, a condition that is also referred to as muscle contraction headache. It occurs as a result of a stressful situation, such as activities that cause the individual stress and anxiety (psychological and environmental factors). The attack may last from several hours to a number of days. Management of the condition includes analgesics, helping the patient to identify activities that precipitate an attack, physical therapy such as heat application to the head and neck area, and relaxation techniques.

A76   D

Tension headaches tend to occur repeatedly in patients who are prone to develop this syndrome. Females experience this condition to a greater extent than males. It may occur at any age and arises because of prolonged contraction of the head and neck muscles. Arterial vasoconstriction in the brain is associated with the prodromal effects of migraine. The vasoconstriction is followed with vasodilation and inflammation leading to pain associated with a migraine attack.

A77   A

Patients with tension headache complain of mild, dull ache that is steady and usually bilateral and non-throbbing. There is scalp tenderness and tightness. They may have sound intolerance and pain may radiate to occipital and frontal areas and neck.

A78   D

GM should be advised to identify factors that are precipitating her attacks. These could include prolonged posture posing strain on head and neck muscles and activities that induce stress. She could be advised to take up some physical activity that will help her to relax. Specific food consumption has not been established to have a direct effect on the occurrence of tension headache. It has been documented that dietary factors such as consumption of cheese and wine may induce migraine attacks.

A79   B

Drugs that can be used to manage an acute attack include paracetamol, non-steroidal analgesics (NSAIDs) such as ibuprofen and combination products such as co-codamol, which contains paracetamol and codeine. NSAIDs and products consisting of paracetamol with an opioid drug such as the co-codamol combination present a better analgesic profile. NSAIDs are anti-inflammatory and this may help in patients where neck muscle inflammation is prominent.

A80   C

Aspirin should not be recommended to GM if she has a history of gastric irritation or if she is breast-feeding. Irritation of the gastric mucosa leading to erosion and ulceration may occur with administration of aspirin and other NSAIDs; the risk is higher in patients with a history of dyspepsia or a lesion of the gastric mucosa. When used during breast-feeding, aspirin enters breast milk and it is transferred to the infant. Aspirin should be avoided during breast-feeding because there is a risk of Reye's syndrome in the infant. Reye's syndrome is a condition characterised by acute encephalopathy and fatty degeneration of the liver that is associated with the use of aspirin in children. Regular use of aspirin by breast-feeding mothers may impair platelet function in the infant resulting in hypoprothrombinaemia. Aspirin or other NSAIDs should not be recommended if GM had haemophilia, as it increases the risk of bleeding, and if GM had asthma, as hypersensitivity and paroxysmal bronchospasms may be precipitated.

Test 3

Questions

Questions 1–6

Directions: Each group of questions below consists of five lettered headings followed by a list of numbered questions. For each numbered question select the one heading that is most closely related to it. Each heading may be used once, more than once, or not at all.

Questions 1–3 concern the following:

A ☐ phaeochromocytoma
B ☐ Cushing's disease
C ☐ cirrhosis
D ☐ Wilson's disease
E ☐ dysentry

Select, from A to E, which one of the above is associated with:

Q1 abnormal copper metabolism

Q2 accumulation of fat on the face, chest and upper back

Q3 hypersecretion of adrenaline and noradrenaline

Questions 4–6 concern the following:

A ☐ hypernatraemia
B ☐ hyponatraemia
C ☐ hypercalcaemia
D ☐ hypocalcaemia
E ☐ hypokalaemia

Select, from A to E, which one of the above:

Q4   may occur as a result of hyperparathyroidism

Q5   may present with arrhythmias

Q6   predisposes to digoxin toxicity

Questions 7–26

Directions: For each of the questions below, ONE or MORE of the responses is (are) correct. Decide which of the responses is (are) correct. Then choose:

A   ☐ if 1, 2 and 3 are correct
B   ☐ if 1 and 2 only are correct
C   ☐ if 2 and 3 only are correct
D   ☐ if 1 only is correct
E   ☐ if 3 only is correct

Directions summarised				
A	B	C	D	E
1, 2, 3	1, 2 only	2, 3 only	1 only	3 only

Q7   Transdermal fentanyl:

1   ☐ is used for pain relief
2   ☐ contains a pure agonist for μ-opioid receptors
3   ☐ provides long-lasting analgesic effect

Q8   Unexpected fluctuations in dose response in patients receiving warfarin may be attributed to:

1   ❑ changes in vitamin K intake
2   ❑ major changes in intake of salads and vegetables
3   ❑ major changes in alcohol consumption

Q9   Clozapine has an affinity for:

1   ❑ dopamine receptors
2   ❑ serotonin receptors
3   ❑ muscarinic receptors

Q10   Ciclosporin:

1   ❑ has an inhibitory effect on T-lymphocytes
2   ❑ may cause a dose-dependent increase in serum creatinine during the first few weeks of treatment
3   ❑ causes hyperlipidaemia

Q11   When candesartan is started in the older person, recommended monitoring includes:

1   ❑ plasma potassium
2   ❑ bilirubin
3   ❑ blood glucose

Q12   Prostate cancer:

1   ❑ testosterone replacement therapy is the mainstay of treatment
2   ❑ growth is androgen-dependent
3   ❑ may be diagnosed by prostate-specific antigen screening

Q13   Ondansetron:

1   ☐ may be administered with dexamethasone
2   ☐ is the drug of first choice in managing delayed chemotherapy-induced nausea and vomiting
3   ☐ is used prophylactically for motion sickness

Q14   Dose reduction and delays in administration of planned cytotoxic chemotherapy are caused by:

1   ☐ alopecia
2   ☐ extravasation
3   ☐ leucopenia

Q15   Spirometry measures:

1   ☐ forced expiratory volume
2   ☐ forced vital capacity
3   ☐ total lung capacity

Q16   Methicillin-resistant *Staphylococcus aureus*:

1   ☐ is a cause of nosocomial infections
2   ☐ spreading of infection may be reduced by alcohol hand rubs
3   ☐ presents an economic issue to institutions

Q17   Alanine aminotransferase:

1   ☐ is found predominantly in the liver
2   ☐ levels are significantly decreased in viral hepatitis
3   ☐ is never released into the bloodstream

Q18   Aldosterone:

1   ☐ production is regulated primarily by the liver
2   ☐ levels are decreased by low-sodium diets
3   ☐ is produced by the adrenal cortex

Q19   Proteinuria:

1   ☐ is an indicator of renal disease
2   ☐ may be an indicator of pre-eclampsia
3   ☐ 24-h urine specimen collection could be recommended if proteinuria is significant

Q20   Patients with type I diabetes should be advised:

1   ☐ to self-monitor blood glucose
2   ☐ to have access to a source of fast sugars
3   ☐ to avoid participating in sport

Q21   When aspirin is compared with warfarin, it:

1   ☐ decreases platelet aggregation
2   ☐ has higher rates of major haemorrhage
3   ☐ requires the same degree of monitoring

Q22   Patients with gallstone disease:

1   ☐ present with visceral pain in the abdomen
2   ☐ report precipitation of the condition with fatty meals
3   ☐ are referred for a gastroscopy

Q23   Sleep apnoea:

1   ☐ is associated with cessation of breathing for at least 5 minutes during sleep
2   ☐ occurs more commonly in obese patients
3   ☐ presents with snoring

Q24   Potential beneficial effects of cannabis include:

1   ☐ anti-emetic
2   ☐ analgesia
3   ☐ appetite suppressant

Q25 Drugs that may cause hypertension include:

1 ☐ corticosteroids
2 ☐ phenothiazines
3 ☐ alpha-adrenoceptor blockers

Q26 Patients receiving oral iron tablets should be advised:

1 ☐ to take the preparation with food
2 ☐ that stools may be black-coloured
3 ☐ to rinse their mouth after drug administration

Questions 27–80

Directions: These questions involve cases. Read the case description or patient profile and answer the questions. For questions with one or more correct answers, follow the key given with each question. For the other questions, only one answer is correct – give the corresponding answer.

Questions 27–43 involve the following case:

> SN is a 25-year-old female who is admitted to the emergency department.
>
> PMH asthma
> DH salbutamol inhaler two puffs three times daily
>   beclometasone 200 µg/puff inhaler two puffs twice daily
> PC chest tightness, exhaustion
> O/E pulse >110 bpm
>   respiration rate >25 breaths/minute
> Diagnosis exacerbation of asthma

SN was hospitalised and the following therapy started:
    oxygen 60%
    salbutamol nebuliser 2.5 mg four times daily
    hydrocortisone intravenous 200 mg every 6 h
    cefuroxime intravenous 750 mg every 8 h
    clarithromycin tablets 500 mg twice daily
    beclometasone inhaler two puffs twice daily

Q27   In an asthmatic attack the following condition(s) occur(s)

1   ☐ bronchospasm
2   ☐ increased airways resistance
3   ☐ inflammation

A   ☐ 1, 2, 3
B   ☐ 1, 2 only
C   ☐ 2, 3 only
D   ☐ 1 only
E   ☐ 3 only

Q28   Inflammatory mediators that are released in an asthmatic attack include:

1   ☐ histamine
2   ☐ leukotrienes
3   ☐ prostaglandins

A   ☐ 1, 2, 3
B   ☐ 1, 2 only
C   ☐ 2, 3 only
D   ☐ 1 only
E   ☐ 3 only

Q29 Drugs that may provoke an asthmatic attack in SN include:

1 ☐ diclofenac
2 ☐ atenolol
3 ☐ timolol

A ☐ 1, 2, 3
B ☐ 1, 2 only
C ☐ 2, 3 only
D ☐ 1 only
E ☐ 3 only

Q30 Signs and symptoms in SN of an acute severe asthma attack include:

1 ☐ tachycardia
2 ☐ tachypnoea
3 ☐ exhaustion

A ☐ 1, 2, 3
B ☐ 1, 2 only
C ☐ 2, 3 only
D ☐ 1 only
E ☐ 3 only

Q31 Salbutamol nebuliser is used in combination with oxygen because:

A ☐ it may mask symptom severity
B ☐ aggressive treatment is required
C ☐ the dose is lower than administered by inhaler
D ☐ it may cause hypovolaemia
E ☐ it may cause arterial hypoxaemia

Q32   Parameters that require monitoring in SN include:

1   ❑   urinary flow
2   ❑   blood gases
3   ❑   plasma-potassium concentration

A   ❑   1, 2, 3
B   ❑   1, 2 only
C   ❑   2, 3 only
D   ❑   1 only
E   ❑   3 only

Q33   If SN's condition does not improve after 30 minutes, the following may be added to the drug therapy:

1   ❑   nebulised ipratropium
2   ❑   intravenous aminophylline
3   ❑   nebulised amoxicillin

A   ❑   1, 2, 3
B   ❑   1, 2 only
C   ❑   2, 3 only
D   ❑   1 only
E   ❑   3 only

Q34   Cefuroxime is:

1   ❑   also available for oral administration
2   ❑   active against *Haemophilus influenzae*
3   ❑   highly effective against Gram-negative bacteria

A   ❑   1, 2, 3
B   ❑   1, 2 only
C   ❑   2, 3 only
D   ❑   1 only
E   ❑   3 only

Q35   Clarithromycin:

1   ☐ is a macrolide
2   ☐ achieves lower tissue concentrations than erythromycin
3   ☐ has poor activity against *Haemophilus influenzae*

A   ☐ 1, 2, 3
B   ☐ 1, 2 only
C   ☐ 2, 3 only
D   ☐ 1 only
E   ☐ 3 only

Q36   Intravenous hydrocortisone is indicated in SN:

1   ☐ to avoid anaphylactic shock
2   ☐ for its mineralcorticoid effects
3   ☐ to inhibit the production and release of pro-inflammatory agents

A   ☐ 1, 2, 3
B   ☐ 1, 2 only
C   ☐ 2, 3 only
D   ☐ 1 only
E   ☐ 3 only

After 24 h SN is reviewed and the following changes are made to the drug therapy:
stop hydrocortisone intravenous
start prednisolone tablets 20 mg daily
change frequency of administration of salbutamol nebuliser to three times daily

Q37   Prednisolone:

1   ☐ should replace beclometasone inhaler
2   ☐ suppresses cortisol secretion
3   ☐ has predominantly glucocorticoid activity

A   ☐ 1, 2, 3
B   ☐ 1, 2 only
C   ☐ 2, 3 only
D   ☐ 1 only
E   ☐ 3 only

Q38   When administering prednisolone:

1   ☐ it should be taken after food
2   ☐ enteric-coated formulation is preferred
3   ☐ dose should be divided into twice daily administration

A   ☐ 1, 2, 3
B   ☐ 1, 2 only
C   ☐ 2, 3 only
D   ☐ 1 only
E   ☐ 3 only

Q39   Nebulisers:

1   ☐ are devices producing an aerosol from an aqueous solution
2   ☐ should be washed out to avoid microbial growth
3   ☐ salbutamol injection solution is used to administer salbutamol
     by nebulisation

A   ☐ 1, 2, 3
B   ☐ 1, 2 only
C   ☐ 2, 3 only
D   ☐ 1 only
E   ☐ 3 only

Q40   Beclometasone inhaler:

1   ☐ is more effective than budesonide
2   ☐ may be used to control an attack
3   ☐ may cause oral candidiasis

A   ☐ 1, 2, 3
B   ☐ 1, 2 only
C   ☐ 2, 3 only
D   ☐ 1 only
E   ☐ 3 only

Q41   Long-term inhalation of high doses of beclometasone may predispose patients to:

1   ☐ osteoporosis
2   ☐ hoarseness
3   ☐ hypertension

A   ☐ 1, 2, 3
B   ☐ 1, 2 only
C   ☐ 2, 3 only
D   ☐ 1 only
E   ☐ 3 only

Q42   Salmeterol:

1   ☐ is longer-acting than salbutamol
2   ☐ may be used in combination with beclomethasone
3   ☐ could replace salbutamol use

A   ☐ 1, 2, 3
B   ☐ 1, 2 only
C   ☐ 2, 3 only
D   ☐ 1 only
E   ☐ 3 only

Q43 SN could be counselled on signs indicating exacerbation of the condition. She could be advised to report:

1 ☐ decrease in exercise tolerance
2 ☐ increased requirements for salbutamol inhaler
3 ☐ increasing peak expiratory flow

A ☐ 1, 2, 3
B ☐ 1, 2 only
C ☐ 2, 3 only
D ☐ 1 only
E ☐ 3 only

Questions 44–57 involve the following case:

GL is a 63-year-old obese male who presents with sudden onset of chest pain.

PMH	diabetes
	hypertension
	ischaemic heart disease
	episode of myocardial infarction two years ago
DH	enalapril tablets 20 mg daily
	aspirin enteric-coated tablets 75 mg daily
	furosemide tablets 20 mg daily
	metformin tablets 500 mg daily
	ranitidine tablets 150 mg nocte
PC	sudden onset of chest pain radiating into throat and left arm, patient is sweating and feeling breathless
O/E	pulse rate 140 bpm
Drug treatment added	heparin subcutaneous 6000 units every 6 h
	isosorbide dinitrate injection 5 mg per hour
Diagnosis	acute attack of unstable angina

Q44   Which signs and symptoms in GL suggest an angina attack?

1   ❏ tachycardia
2   ❏ sweating
3   ❏ breathlessness

A   ❏ 1, 2, 3
B   ❏ 1, 2 only
C   ❏ 2, 3 only
D   ❏ 1 only
E   ❏ 3 only

Q45   During an angina attack investigations that are indicated include:

1   ❏ ECG
2   ❏ blood pressure
3   ❏ coronary angiography

A   ❏ 1, 2, 3
B   ❏ 1, 2 only
C   ❏ 2, 3 only
D   ❏ 1 only
E   ❏ 3 only

Q46   In GL the goals of treatment include:

1   ❏ to reduce symptoms
2   ❏ to improve exercise capacity
3   ❏ to reduce the risk of a heart attack

A   ❏ 1, 2, 3
B   ❏ 1, 2 only
C   ❏ 2, 3 only
D   ❏ 1 only
E   ❏ 3 only

Q47 On admission, therapeutic management of GL should aim to:

1 ☐ reduce cardiac oxygen demand
2 ☐ provide antithrombotic therapy
3 ☐ provide antiplatelet therapy

A ☐ 1, 2, 3
B ☐ 1, 2 only
C ☐ 2, 3 only
D ☐ 1 only
E ☐ 3 only

Q48 Isosorbide dinitrate:

1 ☐ is a coronary vasoconstrictor
2 ☐ flushing may occur
3 ☐ patient may complain of throbbing headache

A ☐ 1, 2, 3
B ☐ 1, 2 only
C ☐ 2, 3 only
D ☐ 1 only
E ☐ 3 only

Q49 Heparin:

1 ☐ has a rapid onset of action
2 ☐ has a short duration of action
3 ☐ patient should be monitored for signs of haemorrhage

A ☐ 1, 2, 3
B ☐ 1, 2 only
C ☐ 2, 3 only
D ☐ 1 only
E ☐ 3 only

Q50   If the patient responds to therapy:

1   ☐ isosorbide dinitrate could be switched to oral administration
2   ☐ heparin is stopped after 10 days
3   ☐ aspirin is stopped

A   ☐ 1, 2, 3
B   ☐ 1, 2 only
C   ☐ 2, 3 only
D   ☐ 1 only
E   ☐ 3 only

Q51   Enalapril:

1   ☐ is an ACE inhibitor
2   ☐ is indicated for hypertension in diabetic patients
3   ☐ is used for long-term management of myocardial infarction

A   ☐ 1, 2, 3
B   ☐ 1, 2 only
C   ☐ 2, 3 only
D   ☐ 1 only
E   ☐ 3 only

Q52   Metformin:

1   ☐ does not cause insulin release
2   ☐ may provoke lactic acidosis
3   ☐ requires monitoring of renal function

A   ☐ 1, 2, 3
B   ☐ 1, 2 only
C   ☐ 2, 3 only
D   ☐ 1 only
E   ☐ 3 only

Q53 Metformin:

1 ☐ does not precipitate hypoglycaemia
2 ☐ should be taken with meals
3 ☐ is indicated because GL is obese

A ☐ 1, 2, 3
B ☐ 1, 2 only
C ☐ 2, 3 only
D ☐ 1 only
E ☐ 3 only

Q54 Drugs that are known to cause hyperkalaemia is (are):

1 ☐ enalapril
2 ☐ heparin
3 ☐ furosemide

A ☐ 1, 2, 3
B ☐ 1, 2 only
C ☐ 2, 3 only
D ☐ 1 only
E ☐ 3 only

GL is discharged and in addition to his medication on admission he is started on simvastatin tablets 20 mg at night and glyceryl trinitrate patch.

Q55 With regards to simvastatin, GL should be advised:

1 ☐ to return for monitoring of liver function tests
2 ☐ that this medication is only for short-term until LDL levels normalise
3 ☐ to avoid use of non-steroidal anti-inflammatory drugs

A   ☐   1, 2, 3
B   ☐   1, 2 only
C   ☐   2, 3 only
D   ☐   1 only
E   ☐   3 only

Q56   With regards to the glyceryl trinitrate patch, GL should be advised:

1   ☐   to apply patch on chest wall, upper arm or shoulder
2   ☐   to change daily
3   ☐   to remove at night

A   ☐   1, 2, 3
B   ☐   1, 2 only
C   ☐   2, 3 only
D   ☐   1 only
E   ☐   3 only

Q57   Additional drug therapy that could be suggested for GL for long-term management include:

1   ☐   glyceryl trinitrate spray
2   ☐   digoxin
3   ☐   vasopressin

A   ☐   1, 2, 3
B   ☐   1, 2 only
C   ☐   2, 3 only
D   ☐   1 only
E   ☐   3 only

Questions 58–62 involve the following case:

MG is a 64-year-old male who was admitted to hospital with a stroke. On admission MG was taking nifedipine slow-release tablets 20 mg three times daily and aspirin tablets 75 mg. He has a past history of hypertension.

MG is started on dipyridamole tablets 100 mg three times daily.

Q58   Dipyridamole should:

1   ☐   be administered before food
2   ☐   be used with caution in hypotension
3   ☐   not to be given with aspirin

A   ☐   1, 2, 3
B   ☐   1, 2 only
C   ☐   2, 3 only
D   ☐   1 only
E   ☐   3 only

Q59   Side-effects associated with dipyridamole include:

1   ☐   headache
2   ☐   abdominal distress
3   ☐   hot flushes

A   ☐   1, 2, 3
B   ☐   1, 2 only
C   ☐   2, 3 only
D   ☐   1 only
E   ☐   3 only

Q60   Nifedipine:

1   ❑ commonly precipitates heart failure
2   ❑ is a highly negative inotropic agent
3   ❑ relaxes coronary and peripheral arteries

A   ❑ 1, 2, 3
B   ❑ 1, 2 only
C   ❑ 2, 3 only
D   ❑ 1 only
E   ❑ 3 only

Q61   Modified-release formulations of nifedipine are preferred to prevent:

1   ❑ large variations in blood pressure
2   ❑ reflex tachycardia
3   ❑ decreased effect in patients with short bowel syndrome

A   ❑ 1, 2, 3
B   ❑ 1, 2 only
C   ❑ 2, 3 only
D   ❑ 1 only
E   ❑ 3 only

Q62   Parameters that should be monitored in MG include:

1   ❑ blood pressure
2   ❑ heart rate
3   ❑ signs and symptoms of heart failure

A   ❑ 1, 2, 3
B   ❑ 1, 2 only
C   ❑ 2, 3 only
D   ❑ 1 only
E   ❑ 3 only

Questions 63–65 involve the following case:

GX is an 80-year-old female who lives on her own and is receiving the following medication:

glibenclamide tablets 10 mg am and 15 mg mid-day
isosorbide mononitrate tablets 60 mg daily
aspirin enteric-coated tablets 75 mg daily
perindopril tablets 8 mg daily
calcium tablets 600 mg daily
cod liver oil capsules once daily

Q63 For which of the following drugs is there an alternative drug that is more appropriate for GX?

A ☐ glibenclamide
B ☐ isosorbide mononitrate
C ☐ aspirin
D ☐ perindopril
E ☐ calcium

Q64 Perindopril:

1 ☐ may lead to deterioration of glucose tolerance
2 ☐ dose in GX should be reviewed due to under-dosing
3 ☐ treatment warrants routine renal function tests to be undertaken

A ☐ 1, 2, 3
B ☐ 1, 2 only
C ☐ 2, 3 only
D ☐ 1 only
E ☐ 3 only

Q65 Isosorbide mononitrate:

1 ☐ has a longer halflife than the dinitrate salt
2 ☐ has poor bioavailability after oral administration
3 ☐ is used in hypertension

A ☐ 1, 2, 3
B ☐ 1, 2 only
C ☐ 2, 3 only
D ☐ 1 only
E ☐ 3 only

Questions 66–73 involve the following case:

AV is a 64-year-old female.

PMH   rheumatoid arthritis
DH   methotrexate tablets 15 mg weekly
         folic acid tablets 10 mg weekly
         prednisolone tablets 5 mg daily
         vitamin D and calcium tablets twice daily
         disodium pamidronate injection 90 mg every 3 months

Q66 Rheumatoid arthritis:

1 ☐ is a localised condition
2 ☐ occurs as a consequence of trauma
3 ☐ affects synovial joints

A ☐ 1, 2, 3
B ☐ 1, 2 only
C ☐ 2, 3 only
D ☐ 1 only
E ☐ 3 only

Q67 Onset of rheumatoid arthritis:

1 ☐ is insidious
2 ☐ occurs symmetrically
3 ☐ is polyarticular

A ☐ 1, 2, 3
B ☐ 1, 2 only
C ☐ 2, 3 only
D ☐ 1 only
E ☐ 3 only

Q68 In monitoring effectiveness of treatment for AV, functional factors to be assessed include:

1 ☐ duration of morning stiffness
2 ☐ ability to dress
3 ☐ grip strength

A ☐ 1, 2, 3
B ☐ 1, 2 only
C ☐ 2, 3 only
D ☐ 1 only
E ☐ 3 only

Q69 AV should be monitored for development of:

1 ☐ anaemia
2 ☐ gastric ulceration
3 ☐ elevated creatine kinase

A ☐ 1, 2, 3
B ☐ 1, 2 only
C ☐ 2, 3 only
D ☐ 1 only
E ☐ 3 only

Q70   AV should be advised:

1   ☐ to take methotrexate and folic acid once weekly one day apart

2   ☐ to take prednisolone after food

3   ☐ to report sore throat or fever immediately

A   ☐ 1, 2, 3
B   ☐ 1, 2 only
C   ☐ 2, 3 only
D   ☐ 1 only
E   ☐ 3 only

Q71   AV should undergo regularly investigations for:

1   ☐ full blood count

2   ☐ renal function tests

3   ☐ liver function tests

A   ☐ 1, 2, 3
B   ☐ 1, 2 only
C   ☐ 2, 3 only
D   ☐ 1 only
E   ☐ 3 only

Q72   Disodium pamidronate:

1   ☐ is used in corticosteroid-induced osteoporosis

2   ☐ is only available for parenteral administration

3   ☐ requires monitoring of serum electrolytes

A   ☐ 1, 2, 3
B   ☐ 1, 2 only
C   ☐ 2, 3 only
D   ☐ 1 only
E   ☐ 3 only

Q73   Disease-modifying antirheumatic drugs that act as cytokine inhibitors include:

1   ☐   methotrexate
2   ☐   etanercept
3   ☐   infliximab

A   ☐   1, 2, 3
B   ☐   1, 2 only
C   ☐   2, 3 only
D   ☐   1 only
E   ☐   3 only

Questions 74–80 involve the following case:

MA is a 71-year-old male who was diagnosed with shingles about 3 months ago. During the active phase of the disease MA received famciclovir tablets 250 mg three times daily for 7 days. MA is still complaining of pain in the area although he reports that the rash has now cleared.

Q74   Shingles:

1   ☐   occurs when varicella zoster virus is reactivated from its latent state
2   ☐   involves primarily the dorsal root ganglia
3   ☐   is characterised by vesicular eruptions

A   ☐   1, 2, 3
B   ☐   1, 2 only
C   ☐   2, 3 only
D   ☐   1 only
E   ☐   3 only

Q75 Shingles:

1 ☐ may present with eye involvement
2 ☐ postherpetic neuralgia does not exceed 2 months in duration
3 ☐ pain is characterised by spasms

A ☐ 1, 2, 3
B ☐ 1, 2 only
C ☐ 2, 3 only
D ☐ 1 only
E ☐ 3 only

Q76 Famciclovir:

1 ☐ has a better bioavailability than aciclovir
2 ☐ is a prodrug of penciclovir
3 ☐ lacks intrinsic antiviral activity

A ☐ 1, 2, 3
B ☐ 1, 2 only
C ☐ 2, 3 only
D ☐ 1 only
E ☐ 3 only

Q77 Famciclovir:

1 ☐ should be started immediately in the active phase
2 ☐ is used to minimise risk of postherpetic neuralgia
3 ☐ should be continued until pain disappears

A ☐ 1, 2, 3
B ☐ 1, 2 only
C ☐ 2, 3 only
D ☐ 1 only
E ☐ 3 only

Q78   Side-effects to be expected with famciclovir include:

1   ❑ hypertension
2   ❑ nausea
3   ❑ headache

A   ❑ 1, 2, 3
B   ❑ 1, 2 only
C   ❑ 2, 3 only
D   ❑ 1 only
E   ❑ 3 only

Q79   MA now has:

A   ❑ migrainous neuralgia
B   ❑ postherpetic neuralgia
C   ❑ trigeminal neuralgia
D   ❑ chickenpox
E   ❑ generalised anxiety disorder

Q80   Drugs that could be used to manage the condition of MA include:

1   ❑ ampicillin
2   ❑ ibuprofen
3   ❑ amitriptyline

A   ❑ 1, 2, 3
B   ❑ 1, 2 only
C   ❑ 2, 3 only
D   ❑ 1 only
E   ❑ 3 only

Test 3

Answers

Questions 1-3

An understanding of pathology of disease states is essential to be able to use drug therapy appropriately and rationally. Unwanted effects of medications may have an impact in a particular patient because of concomitant disease states, resulting in deterioration of the condition.

A1   D

Wilson's disease is a rare disorder associated with a decrease in ceruloplasmin, which causes copper to accumulate slowly in the liver and then be released into the circulation where it is taken up by other tissues. It is an inherited disorder. Accumulation of copper in the brain causes tremors, muscle rigidity and speech impairment, whereas its accumulation in erythrocytes leads to haemolysis and haemolytic anaemia.

A2   B

Cushing's disease is a disorder where there is an increased secretion of adrenocortical steroids. This results in accumulation of fat on the face, chest and upper back and leads to the development of oedema, hyperglycaemia, increased gluconeogenesis, muscle weakness and osteoporosis. In women, acne and facial hair growth may occur. The condition is caused by increased amounts of adrenocorticotrophic hormone, which is released from the pituitary.

A3   A

Phaeochromocytoma is a tumour of the chromaffin tissue of the adrenal medulla or sympathetic paraganglia. Its occurrence results in hypersecretion of adrenaline and noradrenaline leading to the development of persistent or intermittent hypertension, headache, palpitations, sweating, hyperglycaemia, syncope, nausea and vomiting.

Questions 4–6

Serum electrolytes are regularly performed in a battery of clinical laboratory tests. A change in the concentration of electrolytes in blood is important information that is required for diagnosis and for patient monitoring.

A4   C

Hypercalcaemia usually occurs as a result of hyperparathyroidism or because of carcinoma. The serum calcium measurement is used to evaluate parathyroid function and calcium metabolism. Hyperparathyroidism leads to increased parathyroid hormone levels, which lead to increased gastrointestinal absorption of calcium, decreased calcium urinary excretion and increased bone resorption. Symptoms of hypercalcaemia include nausea, vomiting, somnolence and coma.

A5   E

Hypokalaemia leads to decreased contractility of smooth, skeletal and cardiac muscle. This predisposes the patient to weakness, paralysis and cardiac arrhythmias.

A6   E

Hypokalaemia increases cardiac muscle sensitivity to digoxin and hence patients are more prone to digoxin toxicity. Patients who are taking digoxin and may be predisposed to hypokalaemia should have their serum potassium levels monitored and potassium supplementation may be required. Digoxin toxicity is manifested by anorexia, nausea, vomiting, diarrhoea, abdominal pain, visual disturbances, headache, confusion, drowsiness, arrhythmias and heart block.

Questions 7–26

A7   A

Fentanyl is a phenylpiperidine derivative and it is a potent opioid analgesic, which is a pure agonist of μ-opioid receptors. Self-adhesive patches releasing fentanyl are used for chronic intractable pain. The transdermal drug delivery system releases the drug for about 72 h. Fentanyl may be given by intramuscular or intravenous injection as an adjunct to anaesthesia.

A8   A

Warfarin is an anticoagulant that acts by reducing the vitamin-K-dependent synthesis of coagulation factors in the liver. Any activity that changes vitamin K concentrations in the body may result in unexpected fluctuations in dose response in patients receiving warfarin. An increase in vitamin K levels through direct vitamin K intake or through an increased intake of salads and vegetables reverses the effect of warfarin. A decrease in consumption leads to a higher anticoagulant effect for the same dose of warfarin as the levels of vitamin K, which oppose its activity, are reduced. Alcohol has a variable effect on warfarin therapy and major changes in consumption may lead to changes in therapeutic outcome.

A9   A

Clozapine is a dibenzodiazepine which is used as an atypical antipsychotic. It has activity as a dopamine-receptor blocker, an antiserotonergic, an antimuscarinic, an alpha-adrenergic blocker, and an antihistamine. It is indicated in schizophrenia. A major disadvantage is that it may precipitate agranulocytosis.

A10   B

Ciclosporin is a calcineurin inhibitor that is used as an immunosuppressant in organ and tissue transplantation. It has a very specific action on T-lymphocytes and little effect on the bone marrow. It inhibits the activation of calcineurin, which is required for the production of lymphokines, including interleukin-2. When treatment is started, kidney function should be monitored for the first few weeks as a dose-dependent increase in serum creatinine and urea may occur.

A11   D

Candesartan is an angiotensin-II receptor antagonist. When candesartan is started in older persons, monitoring of plasma potassium concentration is recommended as hyperkalaemia may occur occasionally. Older people may be more prone to develop this side-effect because of reduced renal function.

A12   C

Prostate cancer is a slowly progressive adenocarcinoma of the prostate gland. It is detected by prostate-specific antigen test and digital rectal examination. The prostate-specific antigen test evaluates the amount of protein produced by the prostate. The concentration of the protein is elevated in patients with cancer or other prostate disease states. Prostate cancer is largely hormone-related and is associated with androgen-dependent growth. Treatment is aimed at androgen depletion and includes use of anti-androgens such as cyproterone and gonadorelin analogues such as goserelin.

A13   D

Ondansetron is a 5-HT$_3$ antagonist which acts as an anti-emetic by blocking serotonergic receptors in the gastrointestinal tract and in the central nervous system. It is used to counteract cytotoxic chemotherapy-induced nausea and vomiting, and in the postoperative nausea and vomiting that can be caused by anaesthetics and opioid analgesics. In the management of chemotherapy-induced nausea and vomiting, ondansetron is used in patients who are receiving highly emetogenic drugs or when other anti-emetics were inadequate for the prevention of acute symptoms. It may be administered in combination with dexamethasone to improve symptom control. Metoclopramide and prochlorperazine are more effective than the 5-HT$_3$ antagonists in the prevention of delayed chemotherapy-induced nausea and vomiting. Ondansetron is not effective for the prophylaxis of motion sickness. In motion sickness the vestibular apparatus in the ear stimulates the vomiting centre in the medulla of the brain, resulting in nausea, pallor, sweating and increased salivation. 5-HT$_3$ antagonists have minimal effects on the vomiting centre. Hyoscine and centrally acting antihistamines such as cinnarizine and dimenhydrinate are used in the prevention of motion sickness.

A14   E

Cytotoxic drugs cause damage to normal cells, particularly where normal cell division is fairly rapid, including hair follicles, resulting in alopecia and bone-marrow suppression. For cytotoxic drugs that are irritant or vesicant, local irritation and inflammation at the administration site may lead to extravasation. Ulceration and necrosis may develop and further dose administration should be undertaken at other sites. When bone-marrow suppression occurs this may result in leucopenia. Its occurrence is a dose-limiting factor as further drug administration has to be delayed until the leucocyte count is normalised. Leucopenia increases the risk of infection. Patients should be advised to report any signs of infection, such as fever, immediately. Colony-stimulating factors such as filgrastim, pegfilgrastim and lenograstim may be used to reduce the duration of neutropenia in patients receiving cytotoxic chemotherapy.

A15   B

In spirometry, the patient is asked to inhale and then to exhale as rapidly as possible into a spirometer, which records the volume of air exiting the lungs.

Forced vital capacity is measured as it is the amount of air that can be moved during maximal inhalation and exhalation. The residual volume is the volume of air that remains in the lungs after maximal expiration and this value together with the forced vital capacity gives the total lung capacity.

A16   A

Methicillin-resistant *Staphylococcus aureus* (MRSA) strains are resistant to a number of antibacterial drugs. They may be sensitive to vancomycin or teicoplanin. MRSA infections usually occur as a hospital-acquired infection (nosocomial infection). Patients with identified MRSA infections are isolated and carers are asked to undertake special precautions to restrain the spread of infections. Using alcohol hand scrubs after handling patients decreases the spread of infection. As management of the condition requires isolation of the cases and use of expensive medications, MRSA infections in an institution represent an economic burden.

A17   D

Alanine aminotransferase (ALT) is an enzyme that is found mainly in the liver with lower amounts also present in the kidneys, heart and skeletal muscle. Its quantification in blood is used to identify hepatocellular diseases of the liver. In liver injury or conditions such as viral hepatitis, ALT levels are increased as it is released into the bloodstream.

A18   E

Aldosterone is a mineralcorticoid hormone which is produced by the adrenal cortex with action in the renal tubule resulting in sodium and water retention and potassium secretion in urine. Production of aldosterone is regulated primarily by the renin–angiotensin system and to a lesser extent by adreno-corticotrophic hormone, sodium and potassium levels. Low serum sodium levels and high potassium levels stimulate aldosterone production.

A19   A

Occurrence of protein in urine (proteinuria) is an indicator of renal disease, as normally protein is not present in urine because it cannot pass through the glomerular membrane in the renal tubules. When the glomerular membrane is damaged, protein such as albumin seeps through the enlarged gaps in the membrane. Urinalysis to identify presence of proteinuria is carried out to detect renal disease and to detect pre-eclampsia in pregnant women. If urinalysis indicates that there is significant proteinuria, a 24-h urine specimen is collected to quantify the protein loss in 24 h.

A20   B

Type I diabetes usually occurs in young people and is characterised by an inability of the beta-cells in the pancreas to produce insulin. Disease management requires insulin replacement using insulin. Patients should be encouraged to undertake self-monitoring of blood glucose so as to avoid changes in blood glucose levels leading to hyperglycaemia or hypoglycaemia. Patients should be advised to lead a normal lifestyle and should be educated on how to recognise the onset of hypoglycaemia. When symptoms of hypoglycaemia such as sweating, tachycardia and hunger occur, the patient is advised to take immediate action by consuming fast sugars such as glucose itself or sweets. Sports and exercise reduces insulin requirements and decreases cardiovascular risk. A lower dose of insulin may be required before and after sports activities.

A21   D

Aspirin is an antiplatelet drug that decreases platelet aggregation, whereas warfarin is an oral anticoagulant that antagonises the effects of vitamin K. Disadvantages of aspirin when it is used for its antiplatelet effects are that it may cause bronchospasm and haemorrhage including gastrointestinal. Occurrence of haemorrhage is much higher with warfarin and for this reason, patients receiving warfarin should have their prothrombin time monitored.

A22   B

Gallstones consist of cholesterol or bile and are usually asymptomatic. During an acute attack patients usually present with biliary colic that is represented with severe, episodic visceral pain in the abdomen. Pain may be precipitated by a large meal. In patients where the gallstones consist mainly of cholesterol, pain is precipitated with meals that have a high-fat content. Presence of gall-stones is confirmed by ultrasound.

A23   C

Sleep apnoea is characterised during sleep by periods of cessation of breathing ranging from 10 seconds to 3 minutes. It results in loud snoring and gasping. It occurs commonly in obese patients and in patients with chronic obstructive pulmonary disease. Patients with sleep apnoea may complain of daytime sleepiness caused by their fragmented sleep at night. Weight loss in obese patients is recommended as a non-pharmacotherapeutic management strategy.

A24   B

Cannabis is in many countries an illegal drug and may not have approval for medicinal use. It has analgesic, muscle relaxant and appetite stimulant effects. It reduces intraocular pressure and has anti-emetic properties. Nabilone is a synthetic cannabinoid that is used for its anti-emetic properties in the manage-ment of cytotoxic chemotherapy-induced nausea and vomiting that are unresponsive to other anti-emetic modalities.

A25   D

Corticosteroids have mineralcorticoid effects that result in sodium and water retention, which leads to hypertension. Phenothiazines, which are used as antipsychotic drugs, have antimuscarinic and alpha-adrenergic blocking effects. They cause antimuscarinic side-effects such as dry mouth, constipation and difficulty with micturition. They may cause hypotension especially in older people. Alpha-adrenoceptor blocking drugs are used in hypertension and in benign prostatic hyperplasia. They block the alpha-adrenoceptor in the sympathetic nervous system causing vasodilation. Side-effects include hypotension, dizziness, vertigo, headache, fatigue, oedema and sleep disturbances.

A26   B

Iron tablets may cause gastrointestinal irritation and patient may complain of nausea and epigastric pain. The occurrence of these side-effects is reduced by advising the patient to take the preparation with food, even though this strategy lowers the absorption of iron. Side-effects may lead to the patient not taking the medication. Administration of iron salts may lead to discoloration of stools.

Questions 27–43

SN is an asthmatic patient who is using, by inhalation, salbutamol, a short-acting beta$_2$ agonist and beclometasone, a corticosteroid. Asthma is a respiratory condition that is characterised by episodes of dyspnoea and wheezing caused by bronchial constriction, coughing and viscous bronchial secretions. Acute asthma attacks when severe may be fatal. On admission, salbutamol is administered by nebuliser and SN is given oxygen. She is started on hydrocortisone intravenously as an anti-inflammatory drug, cefuroxime (second-generation cephalosporin) intravenously and clarithromycin orally (macrolide) as the antibacterials. Beclometasone inhaler therapy is continued.

A27   A

An asthmatic attack may be precipitated by various factors such as allergens (e.g. pollen), foods (for example, tartrazine colorant) and environmental factors (such as cold air, dust and cigarette smoke). Exposure to these factors may lead to bronchospasm which is followed by the development of increased airways resistance and inflammation.

A28   A

In an acute attack there is an increase of eosinophils in the bronchial epithelium releasing proteins and neurotoxins which damage the epithelium. In addition inflammatory cells such as mast cells and basophils release spasmogens such as histamine, leukotrienes, prostaglandins, thromboxane and platelet-activating factor. These result in bronchospasm and oedema, inflammation and airway hyperactivitiy.

A29   A

Drugs that induce bronchospasm may provoke an asthmatic attack in patients with asthma. SN should be advised to avoid using non-steroidal anti-inflammatory drugs (NSAIDs) such as diclofenac as they may provoke an asthma attack. NSAIDs inhibit cyclo-oxygenase resulting in an increased amount of arachidonic acid that is available. A higher arachidonic acid concentration leads to an increased leukotriene production. Beta-adrenoceptor blockers such as atenolol and timolol may also precipitate an asthmatic attack as they block the sympathetic nervous system and hence induce bronchospasm in the bronchial smooth muscle.

A30   A

On examination SN had rapid heart rate (tachycardia). During an acute attack patients suffer from dyspnoea and with increasing severity of the attack they become anxious, which also increases their heart rate. SN also presented tachypnoea with a respiration rate exceeding 20 breaths/minute. This is caused by hyperventilation, which results in patients feeling unable to speak and complete sentences. SN also presented with exhaustion. Severe asthma attacks interfere with patients' sleep because of the distress caused, particularly when the patient is lying down in bed.

A31   E

The aims of treatment for SN are to promote recovery and to prevent further deterioration. Up to 60% oxygen may be used and in fact SN was administered 60% oxygen. In an acute, severe asthma attack, the arterial carbon dioxide is usually decreased. During the severe attack, use of nebuliser solutions of salbutamol may only aggravate hypoxia. SN is receiving oxygen in conjunction with nebulised salbutamol as salbutamol may increase arterial hypoxaemia.

A32   C

As soon as SN is hospitalised, peak expiratory flow rate, blood gases and serum electrolytes should be measured. These parameters should be continuously monitored to assess improvement in the condition. Blood gases are required to assess hypoxia (P_aO_2 <8 kPa) and to evaluate arterial carbon dioxide. During hypoxia, the risk of hypokalaemia is increased and this risk is increased with the administration of salbutamol, which increases cellular potassium uptake.

A33   B

SN has been administered hydrocortisone by intravenous injection which, together with the oxygen and the nebulised salbutamol, is aimed to improve respiration and pulse within 30 minutes. If this is not achieved, ipratropium by nebulisation may be considered. Ipratropium is an antimuscarinic bronchodilator that when administered by nebulisation is very specific for lung tissue and presents minimal side-effects. Use of nebulised solutions of ipratropium are associated with the occurrence of acute angle closure glaucoma caused by ipratropium aerosol coming in contact with the eye. The risk is further increased if it is administered with nebulised salbutamol. Nebulised ipratropium should be avoided in patients with glaucoma and care should be taken to avoid escape of ipratropium aerosol. This can be minimised by using a tightly fitting mask. Intravenous aminophylline is another option as SN has not been administered theophylline. Aminophylline has a different mode of action to salbutamol and ipratropium. As aminophylline is associated with more adverse effects including a higher risk of hypokalaemia, its use should be restricted to attacks where improvement is not achieved with the other lines of treatment. Aminophylline is administered as a slow intravenous bolus dose because it causes venous irritation and rapid bolus doses may precipitate cardiac arrhythmias, profound hypotension and hypokalaemia.

A34   B

Cefuroxime is a second-generation cephalosporin that is active against Gram-positive cocci and against beta-lactamase-producing strains of *Haemophilus influenzae* and *Neisseria gonorrhoeae*. The acetoxyethyl ester of cefuroxime (cefuroxime axetil) is available for oral administration and the dosage regimen in respiratory tract infections is usually 250–500 mg twice daily.

A35   D

Clarithromycin is a macrolide that is derived from erythromycin. Compared with erythromycin, clarithromycin is better absorbed from the gastrointestinal tract, it achieves higher tissue concentrations and has enhanced activity against *Haemophilus influenzae*.

A36   E

Hydrocortisone is a glucocorticoid drug. It stimulates the synthesis of lipocortin, which inhibits the production and release of intrinsic agents that are associated with inflammation such as phospholipase A2, prostaglandins and leukotrienes.

A37   C

Prednisolone is an oral glucocortioid that is given instead of intravenous hydrocortisone. It has predominantly glucocorticoid activity. Systemic administration of glucocorticoids results in suppression of cortisol secretion from the adrenal cortex and prolonged, high-dose therapy may lead to atrophy of the adrenal cortex. As cortisol secretion is greatest in the morning, the dose should be administered in the morning to minimise disturbance in circadian cortisol secretion. Prednisolone dose should be continued until SN is stabilised. Peak expiratory flow rate should be monitored and care should be taken not to precipitate the condition with early withdrawal of oral prednisolone. Depending on the duration of the oral prednisolone therapy, gradual withdrawal may be required to avoid withdrawal symptoms caused by adrenocortical insufficiency.

A38   B

Oral prednisolone may cause dyspepsia and oesophageal and peptic ulceration. Occurrence of these side-effects is reduced by administering the drug after food and by using an enteric-coated formulation.

A39   B

Nebulisers are medical devices that are used to convert a solution to an aerosol. They can deliver higher doses compared with a metered-dose inhaler. They are preferred in patients who have difficulty in using a metered-dose inhaler, and when higher doses are required such as in an acute attack. Nebulisers should be washed out after each use or at least daily to avoid microbial growth and consequent infection. Solutions that are prepared for use in nebulisers should be used. Salbutamol is available as solution for nebulisation.

A40   E

Beclometasone is a corticosteroid that is being administered to SN as a metered-dose inhaler. Beclometasone and budesonide are equally effective in the management of asthma and they are used as prophylactic therapy to reduce airway inflammation. A common side-effect of inhaled corticosteroids is the development of oral candidiasis. This occurs due to deposits of the drug in the oral cavity promoting superinfection with local *Candida* species. SN may be advised to rinse her mouth with water after inhalation so as to decrease onset of oral candidiasis.

A41   B

With long-term inhalation of high doses of beclometasone (greater than 800 μg daily), patients are predisposed to the occurrence of adrenal suppression, osteoporosis, hoarseness and glaucoma.

A42   B

Salmeterol is a long-acting beta$_2$ agonist with a duration of action of about 12 h. Onset of action occurs within 10 to 20 minutes of administration by inhalation but the maximum effect is not achieved until regular administration of successive doses. It cannot replace salbutamol in the relief of an acute asthma attack. It is recommended to be used in combination with an inhaled corticosteroid as life-threatening asthma attacks have been reported following the use of salmeterol without an inhaled corticosteroid.

A43   B

SN should be advised to monitor for signs that indicate an exacerbation of her condition. She should be advised to report any decrease in exercise tolerance, increased requirements for salbutamol inhaler, and any decrease in peak expiratory flow rate immediately so that her medication may be adjusted so as to avoid the development of an acute, severe attack.

Questions 44–57

GL suffers from a history of diabetes, hypertension and ischaemic heart disease. He has a history of a myocardial infarction. On admission GL is taking enalapril (angiotensin-converting enzyme inhibitor), aspirin as an antiplatelet, furosemide (loop diuretic), metformin (biguanide) and ranitidine (H$_2$-receptor antagonist). He is admitted with an acute attack of unstable angina. On admission GL is administered heparin (anticoagulant) and isosorbide dinitrate (nitrate).

A44   A

Ischaemic heart disease may present with symptoms of angina or develop a myocardial infarction. Angina is due to a mismatch in the oxygen supply and oxygen demand of the cardiac muscle. GL is presenting the characteristic symptom of an angina attack, the sudden onset of chest pain radiating into throat and left arm. In addition, he presents breathlessness, tachycardia with a pulse rate of 140 beats per minute which requires immediate correction, and sweating.

A45   B

Diagnosis is based on past medical history and on the presenting symptoms. An electrocardiogram during an attack will confirm diagnosis by indicating an ST-segment depression. Hypertension may occur during an acute attack of angina and it requires correction. Blood pressure should be monitored.

A46   A

In GL the goals of treatment are to reduce the symptoms of chest pain, breathlessness and tachycardia. In the long-term the goal is to improve exercise capacity and limit risk of onset of a myocardial infarction (heart attack). In ischaemic heart disease, as the number of coronary arteries with atherosclerosis and the extent of occlusion increase, the risk of angina and myocardial infarction increases. Long-term management should consider reducing atherosclerotic lesions with coronary angioplasty.

A47 A

During the management of an acute attack of angina, pharmacotherapy is used to reduce oxygen demand and to improve oxygen supply. In GL isosorbide dinitrate is used. By causing dilation of the coronary veins isosorbide dinitrate reduces venous return and results in a reduction of cardiac output. Oxygen supply may be improved by using antithrombotic therapy and antiplatelet therapy. When patients with ischaemic heart disease feel chest pain they are usually advised to use sublingual glyceryl trinitrate or glyceryl trinitrate spray and to take aspirin preferably dispersed in water or chewed for a more immediate drug release compared with swallowing a tablet. A single-dose of aspirin of 150–300 mg should be given as soon as possible after the attack. Patient or carers should inform health professionals what medication the patient has already taken when symptoms of attack started. Heparin is used to decrease platelet aggregation.

A48 C

Isosorbide dinitrate is a coronary vasodilator and side-effects of peripheral vasodilation may occur. These include flushing, throbbing headache, hypotension and dizziness.

A49 A

When heparin is administered by intravenous or subcutaneous injection, it has a rapid onset of action and an average halflife of 1.5 h. There is variability in halflife ranging between 1 to 6 h depending on a number of factors such as renal impairment and liver disease. It carries a risk of bleeding and the patient should be monitored for signs of haemorrhage.

A50 D

Isosorbide dinitrate is initially given intravenously to achieve a fast onset of action and response. Once GL is stabilised, and no chest pain is reported, isosorbide dinitrate is switched to oral administration. This usually requires 24–48 h. Heparin is given to reduce thrombin generation and fibrin formation and unless there are further complications, treatment is continued for about 48 h. Aspirin is used to reduce the incidence of myocardial infarction and GL should continue taking aspirin daily as he was doing before the acute attack.

A51   A

Enalapril is an angiotensin-converting enzyme (ACE) inhibitor that has anti-hypertensive effects. It is an appropriate choice of antihypertensive in GL as ACE inhibitors are preferred drugs in diabetic patients. It is very important that diabetic patients have their blood pressure very well controlled as these patients have multiple risk factors towards the development of cardiovascular disease. Also both long-standing uncontrolled hypertension and diabetes increase the risk of kidney damage. GL had a myocardial infarction two years earlier. ACE inhibitors have a cardioprotective effect in patients at high risk of cardiovascular disease, including those who suffered a myocardial infarction.

A52   A

Metformin is a biguanide which, unlike sulphonylureas, is not associated with weight gain. It is therefore an appropriate antidiabetic for GL who is obese. It increases insulin sensitivity and increases the utilisation of glucose. It does not interfere with insulin release. It may cause lactic acidosis. During treatment metformin causes conversion of glucose to lactate in the intestinal mucosa; lactate is transported to the liver where it is normally metabolised. High plasma concentrations of metformin such as in renal impairment or high lactate concentrations in blood caused by liver disease and alcohol abuse lead to the inability by the liver to clear the lactate. Metformin should not be used in renal impairment, and diabetic patients receiving metformin should have their renal function monitored to exclude renal function deterioration, which may warrant withdrawal of metformin.

A53 A

Metformin increases the use of glucose and increases insulin sensitivity. It is not associated with onset of hypoglycaemia and it does not cause weight gain. To decrease gastrointestinal side-effects such as abdominal discomfort, nausea, diarrhoea and metallic taste, patients are advised to take tablets with meals. Gastrointestinal side-effects are quite common and in some patients lead to the patient not accepting treatment with metformin.

A54 B

ACE inhibitors such as enalapril interfere with the conversion of angiotensin I to angiotensin II. Angiotensin II is a vasoconstrictor and stimulates aldosterone release. As ACE inhibitors prevent the formation of aldosterone, they reduce potassium excretion and may lead to hyperkalaemia. Heparin may also induce hyperkalaemia because it inhibits aldosterone secretion from the adrenal glands. Risk of hyperkalaemia is increased in diabetic patients, in patients with chronic renal failure and in patients taking potassium-sparing diuretics. Furosemide is a loop diuretic that inhibits sodium, potassium and water retention in the kidney and its use may precipitate hypokalaemia.

A55 D

Simvastatin is a statin that is used as a lipid-lowering agent. Use of statins is recommended in patients with ischaemic heart disease to decrease morbidity and mortality. They are used to reduce low-density-lipoprotein cholesterol and slow atherosclerosis. Patient should be advised to follow a diet low in cholesterol in conjunction with long-term statin therapy. Before initiating statins, liver function tests should be carried out, as statins are contraindicated in active liver disease. There is no interaction between statins and non-steroidal anti-inflammatory drugs.

A56   A

Glyceryl trinitrate patches should be applied on chest wall, upper arm or shoulder and replaced daily. For each application, the patch should be placed on a different area. The patch should be removed at night to provide a nitrate-free period. This will reduce development of tolerance to glyceryl trinitrate.

A57   D

GL may be prescribed glyceryl trinitrate spray which can be used for the prophylaxis of angina when onset of symptoms occur. The patient is advised to apply one or two doses under the tongue and close mouth. If there is no response within 10 minutes, the same dose may be repeated. The advantage of the spray over the sublingual tablets is that sublingual tablets have problems of stability which require the patient to discard any tablets remaining after 8 weeks from opening.

Questions 58–62

On admission, MG is taking nifedipine, a calcium-channel blocker and aspirin as an antiplatelet agent. He is admitted with a stroke, a cerebrovascular accident that is occlusion of a cerebral artery by an embolus in the brain or cerebrovascular haemorrhage. The condition leads to ischaemia of the brain tissues. The location and extent of ischaemia have an impact on the sequelae of the attack. Paralysis, speech impairment or death may occur. In MG, hypertension is a major predisposing factor for stroke. Other factors that increase risk of stroke include age, diabetes, transient ischaemic attacks and previous stroke. MG is admitted to hospital to be given support and medical management of the acute phase of the stroke. The use of antiplatelet agents in the management of a non-haemorrhagic stroke is the main line of treatment aimed at preventing formation of thrombi in the arterial vessels. Aspirin is indicated to be used immediately after a non-haemorrhagic cerebrovascular event. Aspirin has antiplatelet effects as it irreversibly inhibits cyclo-oxygenase, which in platelets is responsible for the conversion of arachidonic acid into thromboxane A_2 which is a vasoconstrictor and stimulates platelet aggregation. Dipyridamole may be used in combination with low-dose aspirin to reduce the risk of recurrent stroke.

A58   B

Dipyridamole is an adenosine reuptake inhibitor and a phosphodiesterase inhibitor which has antiplatelet and vasodilating properties. It is given in oral doses of 300–600 mg daily in divided doses. It is incompletely absorbed from the gastrointestinal tract and therefore it should be administered before food. Dipyridamole should be used with caution in patients with hypotension, heart failure, rapidly worsening angina, aortic stenosis and myocardial infarction. It is essential to avoid hypotension, to maintain systemic circulation and to avoid orthostatic changes in patients with an acute stroke, as compromised blood supply to the brain may precipitate degeneration of the condition.

A59   A

The most common side-effects to be expected from dipyridamole are gastrointestinal effects such as nausea, abdominal pain, constipation, dizziness, throbbing headache, hypotension, hot flushes and tachycardia. Risk of occurrence of constipation is higher in hospitalised patients and in patients with limited mobility.

A60   E

Nifedipine is a dihydropyridine calcium-channel blocker. It has predominant activity as a peripheral and coronary arteries vasodilator. As it has minimal effect on cardiac conduction and negative inotropic effect is very low at therapeutic doses, it rarely precipitates heart failure. It is used in the management of hypertension and for the prophylaxis of angina.

A61   B

Nifedipine is rapidly and efficiently absorbed from the gastrointestinal tract but undergoes an extensive first-pass effect. Following oral administration of normal release tablets, it has a halflife of about 2 h. Use of normal-release tablets in the management of hypertension leads to large variations in blood pressure as a three-times-daily dosage regimen would still leave periods during which blood pressure is not controlled. Also, occurrence of reflex tachycardia is higher. Modified-release preparations are preferred and in fact MG was receiving modified-release tablets of 20 mg three times daily. Bioavailability of slow release formulations is lower than conventional tablets.

A62   A

Blood pressure should be monitored in MG. Hypertension should be controlled and development of hypotension avoided. Heart rate and signs and symptoms of heart failure such as oedema should be monitored.

Questions 63–65

GX is receiving glibenclamide (sulphonylurea), isosorbide mononitrate (nitrate), aspirin (antiplatelet), perindopril (angiotensin-converting enzyme inhibitor), calcium supplement and cod liver oil capsules. From this medication review it can be understood that GX is receiving treatment for the management of diabetes and cardiovascular disease. All the medications except for glibenclamide are prescribed as a single daily dose. For isosorbide mononitrate 60 mg slow-release tablet is prescribed.

A63   A

Glibenclamide is a second-generation sulphonylurea that has a duration of effect of 20–29 h but which may be even longer in older people. Its use in GX should be undertaken with care as the risk of hypoglycaemic attacks is higher than other sulphonylureas such as gliclazide and glipizide. Hypo-glycaemia may lead to confusion, unconsciousness and coma if no immediate intake of glucose is taken. This is of concern for GX who lives on her own. According to this medication profile, GX is taking quite a high dose of gliben-clamide. The usual recommended dose of glibenclamide is 5 mg at breakfast to a maximum of 15 mg daily. The dose of glibenclamide and suitability of the drug for GX should be discussed with the prescribing team.

A64   E

An advantage of angiotensin-converting enzyme (ACE) inhibitors such as perindopril is that they do not interfere with glucose tolerance and they can be used as antihypertensive agents or for the management of heart failure in diabetic patients. A maximum daily dose of 8 mg of perindopril may be recom-mended. Deterioration in renal function, which can be monitored by measuring blood urea and creatinine concentrations, may occur, especially in patients who have existing kidney disease and heart failure. Monitoring parameters to be measured in GX should include renal function.

A65   D

Isosorbide mononitrate is an active metabolite of isosorbide dinitrate. Advan-tages over isosorbide dinitrate include a higher bioavailability after oral administration as it does not undergo first-pass hepatic metabolism and a longer halflife. Isosorbide mononitrate is used in the prophylaxis of angina and in congestive heart failure.

Questions 66–73

AV is receiving treatment for rheumatoid arthritis. This is a chronic, progress-ive inflammatory disease that leads to articular and extra-articular symptoms which present significant morbidity to the patient. The condition reduces life expectancy. AV is receiving a disease-modifying antirheumatic drug, methotrexate and prednisolone, as an anti-inflammatory agent. She is also receiving folic acid, calcium and vitamin D supplements and disodium pamidronate, which is a biphosphonate. In rheumatoid arthritis, aims of treatment are to decrease disease progression, limit morbidity and decrease occurrence of flare-ups.

A66   E

Rheumatoid arthritis is associated with inflammation of the synovial membrane of different joints. It is not a localised condition and affects different joints commonly in the hands, wrists, knees, feet and shoulders. Trigger factors are not clear but there is evidence that the condition is immune-mediated.

A67   A

There is great inter-patient variation in the course of the disease. Onset is insidious and the disease usually presents initially with non-specific symptoms such as fatigue, malaise, diffuse musculoskeletal pain and stiffness. Characteristically, at onset the patient presents with symmetrical small-joint polyarthritis in the hands, wrists and feet. Diagnostic criteria for rheumatoid arthritis include presence of morning stiffness, presence of arthritis in three or more joints, symmetrical involvement, rheumatoid nodules, serum rheumatoid factor and radiographic changes.

A68   A

As rheumatoid arthritis progresses, morning stiffness becomes prolonged and more disabling, interfering with patient's daily activities. When assessing outcomes of therapy, functional assessment and impact on the patient's lifestyle should be considered. Factors to be taken into account include duration of morning stiffness, the patient's ability to dress and carry out daily activities, and grip strength.

A69   B

As rheumatoid arthritis is a chronic inflammatory disease, patients may develop anaemia. This occurs because of reduced erythropoiesis during inflammatory disease. The use of prednisolone for long periods may cause peptic ulceration with perforation leading to gastrointestinal bleeding, which may be another cause for anaemia. Methotrexate may also cause intestinal ulceration and bleeding. Development of signs and symptoms of gastric irritation and ulceration should be monitored and AV should be asked to report any gastrointestinal effects. Measurement of creatine kinase (CK) is indicated in the diagnosis of myocardial infarction, neurological or skeletal muscle disease.

A70   A

In AV methotrexate is prescribed as a weekly dose of 15 mg. It is very important to advise AV about proper administration of the drug and the pharmacist should ensure that the patient has understood the dosage regimen. Fatalities may occur if patients inadvertently take the drug at this dose daily. Methotrexate is considered to be a first-line drug in the management of rheumatoid arthritis and the usual maximum dose is 15 mg once a week. AV is given folic acid to reduce nausea and stomatitis, which may be side-effects of methotrexate. It is also given as a once weekly dose, and to aid compliance the patient is advised to take folic acid the day after methotrexate administration. Methotrexate may cause bone marrow suppression and therefore patients are more prone to develop infections. AV should be advised to report immediately any signs of an infection such as sore throat or fever. Methotrexate may also cause pulmonary toxicity, and patients should be asked to report cough and dyspnoea. Bone marrow suppression may be further increased by long-term administration of prednisolone, a glucocorticoid. As both methotrexate and prednisolone may cause gastrointestinal ulceration, AV should be advised to take tablets after food.

A71   A

As methotrexate may cause bone marrow suppression, the patient should have a full blood count, including differential white cell count, regularly. If significant leucopenia or thrombocytopenia occurs, treatment should be stopped as the condition may be fatal. Renal function should also be monitored, as the use of methotrexate in moderate or severe renal impairment is not recommended. Methotrexate may cause liver cirrhosis, and liver function tests should be carried out regularly. AV should be advised to avoid alcohol to lower her risk of hepatic damage.

A72   A

Disodium pamidronate is a biphosphonate that may be used in the prophylaxis and treatment of osteoporosis and corticosteroid-induced osteoporosis. AV is receiving prednisolone as a long-term medication to suppress symptoms of the disease. Discontinuation of treatment may lead to flare-ups of the condition. Long-term use of corticosteroids is associated with onset of osteoporosis, diabetes and hypertension. AV is a post-menopausal woman who is at a higher risk of developing osteoporosis, compared with the normal female cohort group, as she is also receiving prednisolone long-term therapy. In AV disodium pamidronate is used to counteract corticosteroid-induced osteoporosis. A disadvantage of disodium pamidronate is that it is only available for slow intravenous infusion, which is given every 3 months, requiring the patient to be hospitalised for about 3 h. Its use may lead to hypocalcaemia and serum electrolytes should be monitored. Other biphosphonates such as alendronic acid and risedronate, which are available as once weekly oral formulations, may be considered as an alternative. AV is receiving calcium and vitamin D supplementation to prevent hypocalcaemia and as bone supplements in the management of osteoporosis.

A73   C

Disease-modifying antirheumatic drugs include cytokine inhibitors such as etanercept and infliximab. These two drugs inhibit tumour necrosis factor, which is an inflammatory mediator that contributes to synovitis and joint destruction in rheumatoid arthritis. Both drugs are available for parenteral administration. They are recommended for use in rheumatoid arthritis when other disease-modifying antirheumatic drugs have failed to achieve symptom control. As they have been associated with the onset of severe infections, including tuberculosis, patients should be evaluated for tuberculosis before treatment and asked to report any signs of infection.

Questions 74–80

MA suffered an acute attack of shingles, which is caused by the virus herpes zoster. The condition is associated with a unilateral rash and the patient complains of pain which may continue after the rash has disappeared, leading to postherpetic neuralgia.

A74   A

Shingles occurs as a result of reactivation of the varicella zoster virus that is dormant in the nuclear DNA of dorsal root ganglia. Reactivation of the virus may occur as a result of a reduction of the host immunity. The virus tracks down the nerve axon to cause a skin infection in the area innervated by the sensory nerve and this is characterised by vesicular eruptions.

A75   D

Shingles usually occurs along the thorax, head and neck and lumbosacral area. Eye or ear involvement may occur and this requires referral of the patient to a specialist to limit long-term damage. Postherpetic neuralgia may develop as a chronic painful condition that may last from months to years after the acute phase of shingles. Postherpetic neuralgia presents with severe, continuous, burning pain.

A76   A

Famciclovir is a prodrug of penciclovir. Famciclovir is rapidly absorbed from the gastrointestinal tract following oral administration and it is converted to penciclovir. Penciclovir itself is poorly absorbed from the gastrointestinal tract. Famciclovir has better bioavailability (70%) compared with aciclovir (30%) after oral administration. For this reason famciclovir and valaciclovir, which is a prodrug of aciclovir, require less frequent dosing compared with aciclovir in the management of shingles. MA was receiving famciclovir 250 mg tablets three times daily during the acute phase.

A77   B

Use of antiviral drugs such as famciclovir at the onset of the acute phase reduces the risk of postherpetic neuralgia. Famciclovir should be continued for 7 days. MA has finished the treatment with famciclovir.

A78   C

Side-effects associated with famciclovir are rare and these include nausea, headache, confusion, vomiting, jaundice, dizziness, drowsiness, hallucinations, rash and pruritus.

A79   B

As the rash has disappeared and MA is still feeling pain, he has developed postherpetic neuralgia. Occurrence of severe pain during the acute phase is associated with an increased likelihood that the patient develops postherpetic neuralgia.

A80   C

Drugs which could be recommended for MA include analgesics such as non-steroidal anti-inflammatory drugs, for example, ibuprofen. They may provide some pain relief. Patient should be advised to take medication with food and they should not be used if MA has a history of peptic ulcer disease or asthma or if he is on anticoagulant therapy. Tricyclic antidepressants such as amitriptyline may be used as an adjunct analgesic drug that is administered at night to alleviate pain and also induce sedation. If the patient still complains of pain, then anticonvulsants such as carbamazepine and gabapentin may be used.

Test 4

Questions

Questions 1–6

Directions: Each group of questions below consists of five lettered headings followed by a list of numbered questions. For each numbered question select the one heading that is most closely related to it. Each heading may be used once, more than once, or not at all.

Questions 1–3 concern the following:

A ☐ ophthalmoscope
B ☐ otoscope
C ☐ stethoscope
D ☐ sphygmomanometer
E ☐ reflex hammer

Select, from A to E, which one of the above is used:

Q1 to investigate retinopathy

Q2 to assess breath sounds

Q3 to test deep tendon reflexes

Questions 4–6 concern the following:

A ☐ gonadotrophin-releasing hormone
B ☐ C peptide
C ☐ troponin I
D ☐ prolactin
E ☐ human chorionic gonadotrophin

Select, from A to E, which one of the above:

Q4   is produced by the placenta

Q5   is released from the beta cells of the pancreas

Q6   is released from the anterior pituitary gland

Questions 7–26

Directions: For each of the questions below, ONE or MORE of the responses is (are) correct. Decide which of the responses is (are) correct. Then choose:

A   ☐ if 1, 2 and 3 are correct
B   ☐ if 1 and 2 only are correct
C   ☐ if 2 and 3 only are correct
D   ☐ if 1 only is correct
E   ☐ if 3 only is correct

Directions summarised				
A	B	C	D	E
1, 2, 3	1, 2 only	2, 3 only	1 only	3 only

Q7   Creatine kinase (CK):

1   ☐ is found in skeletal muscle
2   ☐ isoenzyme fractions are used to identify the type of tissue damaged
3   ☐ CK-MB are detected in blood within 3–5 h of a myocardial infarction

Q8   Auscultation of bowel sounds:

1   ☐ is usually carried out postoperatively
2   ☐ always requires a stethoscope
3   ☐ when positive, indicates absence of peristalsis

Q9   A complete blood count consists of:

1   ☐ haemoglobin quantification
2   ☐ white blood cells count
3   ☐ blood crossmatching

Q10   The erythrocyte sedimentation rate:

1   ☐ is a non-specific indicator of inflammation
2   ☐ measures the rate at which red blood cells settle out of mixed venous blood
3   ☐ determination is based on protein electrophoresis

Q11   Gastro-oesophageal reflux disease may be associated with:

1   ☐ acid regurgitation
2   ☐ dysphagia
3   ☐ stricture formation

Q12   Patients using co-magaldrox preparations should be advised:

1   ☐ not to take product at the same time as other drugs, except for enteric-coated tablets
2   ☐ to take the preparation after meals
3   ☐ that the product may be taken as required

Q13   Patients should be advised to avoid direct sunlight when taking:

1   ☐ gliclazide
2   ☐ clarithromycin
3   ☐ amiodarone

Q14   Human immunoglobulins:

1   ❏ are prepared from pooled human plasma or serum
2   ❏ are tested for hepatitis B surface antigen
3   ❏ are less likely to be associated with hypersensitivity reactions
     compared with antisera

Q15   Glue ear:

1   ❏ may occur in association with inflammation of the sinuses
2   ❏ may result in long-term hearing impairment
3   ❏ requires systemic antibacterial treatment as the usual line of
     action

Q16   In chronic hepatitis C:

1   ❏ peginterferon is preferred to interferon as pegylation
     increases the persistence of interferon in blood
2   ❏ liver damage may occur, requiring a liver transplant to
     prevent death from cirrhosis
3   ❏ the aim of treatment is to achieve clearance of the virus
     which is sustained for at least 1 month after treatment has
     stopped

Q17   It is recommended that long-term therapy for patients presenting with
     stroke should consider use of:

1   ❏ ACE inhibitor
2   ❏ aspirin
3   ❏ statin

Q18   In patients with stage III (Duke's C) colon cancer, the choice of adjuvant
     chemotherapy should take into account:

1   ❏ the side-effect profile of the drugs
2   ❏ the method of administration
3   ❏ the patient's lifestyle

Q19 The use of calcium supplementation to reduce risk of fractures:

1 ❑ is associated with poor compliance because of the need for sustained treatment

2 ❑ may be combined with vitamin D supplementation

3 ❑ consists of calcium lactate as it is the only salt that can be used for oral administration

Q20 Myopia:

1 ❑ results in light rays being focused behind the retina

2 ❑ can be corrected by using concave lenses for spectacles or contact lenses

3 ❑ occurs when the person cannot clearly see an object that is more than 1 metre from the eye

Q21 Patients who are following a low-fat diet should be advised to:

1 ❑ increase their fibre intake

2 ❑ reduce their intake of saturated fats

3 ❑ eliminate their intake of polyunsaturates

Q22 Patients with atopic eczema should be advised:

1 ❑ to avoid frequent bathing

2 ❑ to avoid scratching the area involved

3 ❑ that the skin is more susceptible to microbial colonisation

Q23 Measurement of drug plasma concentrations is recommended when patients are started on:

1 ❑ phenytoin

2 ❑ cancer chemotherapy

3 ❑ alteplase

Q24 People with irritable bowel syndrome may complain of:

1 ☐ a negative effect on their social life
2 ☐ abdominal pain
3 ☐ gastro-oesophageal reflux

Q25 Immunosuppressive agents that may be used after kidney transplantation include:

1 ☐ azathioprine
2 ☐ ciclosporin
3 ☐ prednisolone

Q26 Anaemia in cancer patients:

1 ☐ often develops insiduously
2 ☐ may be corrected with the use of erythropoietin
3 ☐ is always due to cancer chemotherapy

Questions 27–80

Directions: These questions involve cases. Read the case description or patient profile and answer the questions. For each of the questions below, ONE or MORE of the responses is (are) correct. Decide which of the responses is (are) correct. Then choose:

A ☐ if 1, 2 and 3 are correct
B ☐ if 1 and 2 only are correct
C ☐ if 2 and 3 only are correct
D ☐ if 1 only is correct
E ☐ if 3 only is correct

Directions summarised				
A	B	C	D	E
1, 2, 3	1, 2 only	2, 3 only	1 only	3 only

Questions 27–34 involve the following case:

LJ is a 66-year-old female who was admitted to the medical ward for the management of atrial fibrillation.

PMH   hypertension, asthma
DH   potassium chloride one tablet daily
      bendroflumethiazide 5 mg daily
      warfarin 3 mg daily
O/E   blood pressure 210/95 mmHg

On hospitalisation, digoxin was started at a loading dose of 0.25 mg daily and perindopril 2 mg nocte.

Q27   Atrial fibrillation:

1   ☐ may be caused by hypertension
2   ☐ denote a fast, chaotic rhythm originating from multiple foci in the atria
3   ☐ is associated with ventricular premature beats

Q28   Drugs that could alter QT interval in an ECG include:

1   ☐ amitriptyline
2   ☐ lithium
3   ☐ fluoxetine

Q29   Atrial fibrillation increases the risk of:

    1   ☐ stroke

    2   ☐ heart failure

    3   ☐ hypertension

Q30   The reasons why digoxin was preferred to other options are:

    1   ☐ beta-adrenoceptors should be avoided because of the history of asthma

    2   ☐ digoxin slows ventricular response in atrial fibrillation

    3   ☐ it also has a hypotensive effect

Q31   Digoxin should be used with caution in:

    1   ☐ elderly patients

    2   ☐ renal impairment

    3   ☐ recent infarction

Q32   Parameters that should be monitored include:

    1   ☐ serum potassium levels

    2   ☐ plasma digoxin concentration

    3   ☐ ventricular rate at rest

Q33   A low dose of perindopril is used because:

    1   ☐ the patient is elderly

    2   ☐ the risk of dehydration is very high

    3   ☐ perindopril is being used as a prophylactic of cardiovascular events

Q34   The medication review once the patient is stabilised should assess the need for continuation of treatment with:

    1   ☐ potassium supplementation

    2   ☐ perindopril

    3   ☐ warfarin

Questions 35–43 involve the following case:

AX, a 72-year-old male was referred to casualty because of a 3-week history of fever and painful joints. He presents with an increased swelling and warmth in hands, wrists and ankles. The patient was being well controlled on methotrexate 15 mg weekly up to the last visit to the rheumatology clinic four weeks ago.

PMH   rheumatoid arthritis
           peptic ulceration
           colonic polyps
DH   fluvastatin 20 mg nocte
           methotrexate 15 mg weekly
           folic acid 10 mg weekly
           paracetamol 1 g 8 hourly/prn
Drug allergies   leflunomide
           gold injections caused reversible renal impairment
SH   lives with wife, °alcohol, °smoking
O/E   swollen, warm, tender R and L hand, R and L wrist, R and L ankles
           nodules on left elbow
           bilateral metatarsalgia
           multiple metatarsal deformities
           spindling of digits and wasting of small muscle of hand
Investigations   ECG: normal
           CXR: normal
           random blood glucose: 7.8 mmol/l (<7.8 mmol/l)
           temperature: 37°C
           WBC: 9.7×10^9/l ($5–10.0 \times 10^9$/l)
           RBC: 3.9×10^{12}/l ($4.4–5.8 \times 10^{12}$/l)
           platelets: 250×10^9/l ($150–400 \times 10^9$/l)
           U&Es: normal
Impression   rheumatoid arthritis flare-up

On admission to the ward AX was administered methlyprednisolone 500 mg by slow intravenous infusion for one day.

Q35 The aim(s) of treatment in rheumatoid arthritis is (are):

1 ☐ to preserve functional ability
2 ☐ to prevent osteoporosis
3 ☐ to prevent hyperuricaemia

Q36 Biochemical investigations to monitor AX include:

1 ☐ C-reactive protein
2 ☐ erythrocyte sedimentation rate
3 ☐ rheumatoid factor

Q37 The use of methylprednisolone in AX:

1 ☐ results in suppression of cytokines
2 ☐ presents a rapid improvement in symptoms
3 ☐ should be continued orally for a few months

Q38 Disadvantages of using methylprednisolone in AX include:

1 ☐ his past history of peptic ulceration
2 ☐ concomitant administration with fluvastatin
3 ☐ his allergy to leflunomide

Q39 Compared with prednisolone, methylprednisolone:

1 ☐ has greater glucocorticoid activity
2 ☐ has less mineralcorticoid activity
3 ☐ is gastro-labile

Q40 The interpretation of the results of the blood glucose tests for AX:

1 ☐ requires information on food intake for the past 16 h
2 ☐ indicates hyperglycaemia
3 ☐ may be affected by methylprednisolone therapy

Q41   In the long-term, drugs that could be considered as additional treatment to methotrexate for the management of rheumatoid arthritis in AX include:

1   ❑   infliximab
2   ❑   etanercept
3   ❑   doxorubicin

Q42   Common problems associated with methotrexate therapy in rheumatoid arthritis include:

1   ❑   inadvertent daily drug administration
2   ❑   nausea and vomiting
3   ❑   bone marrow suppression

Q43   AX is receiving folic acid:

1   ❑   to prevent megaloblastic anaemia
2   ❑   to augment the effectiveness of methotrexate
3   ❑   to reduce the occurrence of stomatitis from methotrexate

Questions 44–47 involve the following case:

MB is a 55-year-old male who presented to the emergency department complaining of palpitations. His blood pressure was found to be 150/110 mmHg. Patient stated that he was previously admitted to hospital with hypertension. On questioning he said that he was on moxonidine 200 µg twice daily but that he had stopped the medication because he had run out of tablets. The patient said that he was used to having high blood pressure but never suffered from palpitations.

Q44   Moxonidine:

1   ❑   is a centrally acting antihypertensive drug
2   ❑   acts on the imidazoline receptors
3   ❑   should not be used in patients hypersensitive to ACE inhibitors

Q45   Other drugs that have a similar mode of action to moxonidine include:

1   ❑ methyldopa
2   ❑ doxazosin
3   ❑ hydralazine

Q46   Clinical presentation of MB is probably caused by:

1   ❑ heart failure
2   ❑ stroke
3   ❑ abrupt withdrawal of moxonidine

Q47   The assessment of end-organ damage from hypertension includes:

1   ❑ evaluating prostatic hypertrophy
2   ❑ examination of the optic fundi
3   ❑ carrying out an ECG

Questions 48–52 involve the following case:

RB is a 30-year-old female with a history of systemic sclerosis admitted for treatment of acute Raynaud's phenomenon.

PMH   9-year history of Raynaud's disease with discoloration and cyanosis of fingers on exposure to cold temperatures.

SH   married, ° children, ° alcohol, smoker, works as a salesperson

DH   pentoxifylline 400 mg daily
nifedipine 20 mg daily

O/E   well hydrated
° fever, ° chills, ° rigors
° cough, ° sputum, ° chest pain, ° palpitations
° anorexia, ° weight loss
BP: 117/75 mmHg
pulse: 60 bpm

Left index fingertip is swollen and red, mild tenderness and loose nail. The thumb is swollen and tender. There is mild erythema with a small amount of clear discharge beneath the nail fold.

Q48 The management plan for RB should include:

1 ☐ diclofenac suppositories
2 ☐ vancomycin po
3 ☐ co-amoxiclav intravenous therapy

Q49 Pentoxifylline:

1 ☐ acts as a vasodilator
2 ☐ may cause hypotension
3 ☐ should not be used for longer than 6 weeks

Q50 RB should be advised:

1 ☐ to avoid exposure to cold
2 ☐ to stop smoking
3 ☐ that the condition is precipitated by exercise

Q51 Drugs that should be used with caution or avoided in RB include:

1 ☐ atenolol
2 ☐ codeine
3 ☐ promethazine

Q52 Nifedipine:

1 ☐ has more influence on the myocardium than on peripheral vessels compared with verapamil
2 ☐ should not be administered as a modified-release formulation in the management of Raynaud's phenomenon
3 ☐ reduces frequency and severity of vasospastic effects in Raynaud's phenomenon

Questions 53–59 involve the following case:

FG is an 83-year-old female presenting with a sudden episode of shortness of breath and retrosternal chest pain. She said she was having occasional cough and whitish sputum. Symptoms were accompanied with cold sweat, slight nausea but no vomiting. No abdominal pain and no fever have been reported.

PMH diabetes mellitus controlled by diet, hypertension, congestive heart failure, depression

DH paroxetine 20 mg daily
potassium chloride 600 mg tds
verapamil 40 mg tds
dipyridamole 25 mg daily
bumetanide 1 mg daily
multivitamins one tablet daily

SH lives with elderly sister

O/E BP: 148/90 mmHg
pulse: 70 bpm
temperature: 35.5°C
chest: creps up to apices bilaterally
abdomen: soft, non-tender
° oedema, ° DVT

Investigations ECG: ST depression and T wave flattening
CXR: cardiomegaly
Na 136 (135–145 mmol/l)
K 3.2 (3.5–5.0 mmol/l)
CK 274 (<175 U/l)
urea 9.5 (3.0–8.0 mmol/l)
creatinine 94 (50–110 µmol/l)
WBC: 16×10^9 ($5–10 \times 10^9$ /l)
glucose 19.1 mmol/l (<7.8 mmol/l)

Impression pulmonary oedema secondary to myocardial infarction, chest infection

Q53   On admission treatment that should be started includes:

1   ☐ insulin
2   ☐ isosorbide dinitrate injections
3   ☐ aspirin 75 mg po

Q54   Possible adjustments to FG's current treatment include:

1   ☐ review dose of potassium chloride supplement
2   ☐ switch bumetanide to intravenous therapy
3   ☐ stop verapamil

Q55   Oxygen therapy is started in the A&E department:

1   ☐ to provide initial support
2   ☐ at a concentration of 35%
3   ☐ should be administered using a nasal cannula

Q56   Paroxetine:

1   ☐ is more effective than tricyclic antidepressants
2   ☐ has a similar chemical structure to fluoxetine
3   ☐ may cause movement disorders as side-effects

Q57   Dipyridamole:

1   ☐ is a phosphodiesterase inhibitor
2   ☐ should be used with caution in rapidly worsening angina
3   ☐ is commonly associated with bleeding disorders

Q58   Cardiomegaly:

1   ☐ occurs to accommodate increased ventricular load
2   ☐ leads to pulmonary congestion
2   ☐ may present with tachycardia

Q59   Drugs that could cause hypotension in the patient include:

1   ☐ bumetanide
2   ☐ dipyridamole
3   ☐ paroxetine

Questions 60–66 involve the following case:

AP is a 71-year-old female with a history of hypertension, diabetes mellitus, ischaemic heart disease and congestive heart failure. A year ago she had a myocardial infarction.

Patient presents with 3-day history of central compressive chest pain radiating to epigastrum that is associated with sweating and belching. No nausea, vomiting, shortness of breath and palpitations are reported. Pain started at rest, occurs on and off and worsens on exertion, especially when going upstairs. Patient claims the pain is very similar to previous myocardial infarction pain episode.

ECG showed T wave inversion. CK was 265 (<175 U/l).

SH   married, lives with husband. Non-smoker, no alcohol. Father died at 58 and had a history of diabetes and ischaemic heart disease, mother was diabetic.

O/E   heart sounds normal
chest X-ray normal
few bibasal creps
abdomen is soft, non-tender
no left leg calf tenderness
mild pitting oedema
no signs of DVT
BP: 130/80 mmHg
pulse 68 bpm

DH   candesartan 16 mg daily
clopidrogel 75 mg daily
isosorbide mononitrate 60 mg daily
fluvastatin 80 mg nocte

amlodipine 10 mg daily
carvedilol 6.25 mg bd
bumetanide 1 mg tds
isophane insulin (human) 32 units am and 12 units pm
Impression   unstable angina

Q60   Carvedilol:

1   ☐ has an arteriolar vasodilating action
2   ☐ reduces mortality in heart failure
3   ☐ is more water soluble than atenolol

Q61   Potential side-effects that AP may present include:

1   ☐ postural hypotension
2   ☐ flushing
3   ☐ shortness of breath

Q62   Candesartan:

1   ☐ inhibits breakdown of bradykinin
2   ☐ dose should be administered in divided doses
3   ☐ should be used with caution in renal artery stenosis

Q63   As regards diabetes management:

1   ☐ insulin used is an intermediate-acting preparation
2   ☐ AP should be advised to avoid episodes of hypoglycaemia
3   ☐ insulin requirements decrease during anginal attacks

Q64   Isosorbide mononitrate:

1   ☐ modified-release formulations are preferred
2   ☐ is metabolised to isosorbide dinitrate
3   ☐ increases venous return

Q65 Fluvastatin:

1 ☐ patient should be advised to report muscle pain promptly
2 ☐ a therapeutic alternative is simvastatin 80 mg daily
3 ☐ a complete blood count should be carried out before starting treatment

Q66 The management of unstable angina includes:

1 ☐ clopidrogel
2 ☐ heparin
3 ☐ complete bed rest

Questions 67–70 involve the following case:

KB, a 36-year-old female, presents with complaints of dysuria, urinary urgency and increased frequency.

Q67 Possible diagnoses include:

1 ☐ cystitis
2 ☐ acute pyelonephritis
3 ☐ vulvovaginitis

Q68 The patient should be asked:

1 ☐ about presence of fever
2 ☐ to undertake a urinalysis
3 ☐ to present mid-stream sampling for culturing

Q69 The patient should be advised to:

1 ☐ drink lots of fluid
2 ☐ use potassium citrate salts
3 ☐ use a high dose of ibuprofen

Q70 Anti-infectives that could be recommended include:

1 ☐ co-amoxiclav
2 ☐ cefuroxime
3 ☐ flucloxacillin

Questions 71–75 involve the following case:

SC, a 34-year-old female in her first month of pregnancy, was diagnosed as having a blood pressure of 140/100 mmHg. Full examination showed that all other investigations were normal. She was started on labetalol 100 mg daily.

Q71 The diagnosis indicates:

1 ☐ the probability that hypertension was pre-existing
2 ☐ a higher risk of pre-eclampsia
3 ☐ that hypertension is due to secondary causes

Q72 The patient requires frequent monitoring of:

1 ☐ blood pressure
2 ☐ urinalysis
3 ☐ fetal growth

Q73 During pregnancy, antihypertensives that should be avoided or used with caution include:

1 ☐ thiazide diuretics, as they may cause neonatal thrombocytopenia
2 ☐ ACE inhibitors, as they may affect renal function
3 ☐ beta-blockers, as they may cause intrauterine growth restriction

Q74   Drugs that could be used instead of labetalol include:

1   ☐ furosemide
2   ☐ candesartan
3   ☐ methyldopa

Q75   Labetalol:

1   ☐ acts as a competitive antagonist to alpha and beta receptors in the sympathetic nervous system
2   ☐ structure consists of two optical centres
3   ☐ activity at the alpha receptors results in vasoconstriction

Questions 76–80 involve the following case:

HG, a 46-year-old female presents with complaints of a troublesome cough at night, nasal congestion and nasal itchiness. The symptoms have been present for the past weeks. She states that she has nasal allergy most of the time but now the condition seems to have deteriorated.

She has been using oxymetazoline spray two puffs three times a day for the past two weeks. She has tried to use some tablets previously but has stopped them.

Q76   The patient:

1   ☐ probably has perennial allergic rhinitis
2   ☐ may be allergic to house dust
3   ☐ has a viral infection

Q77   Oxymetazoline:

1   ☐ is effective against nasal congestion
2   ☐ the patient should be advised to stop using it
3   ☐ is also available as an oral formulation

Q78 Desloratidine:

1   ❏ is indicated in this patient on a long-term basis
2   ❏ is available as a nasal spray
3   ❏ oral dosage form requires administration three times daily

Q79 Budesonide:

1   ❏ should be used in the form of tablets
2   ❏ is only available as a nasal spray
3   ❏ is used in the prophylaxis of asthma

Q80 Patient should be advised:

1   ❏ to avoid walking in gardens
2   ❏ to regularly use products to eradicate house dust mites
3   ❏ that the condition could easily develop into cough with blood
         in sputum

Test 4

Answers

Questions 1–3

Medical devices are used for the diagnosis and monitoring of diseases. Accuracy and reliability of the device may vary and reflect on the product's costs. Specifications for medical devices may depend on their intended use.

A1　A

An ophthalmoscope is used to examine the fundus of the eye, which consists of the retina, retinal vessels, sclera, optic disk and choroids. It can be used to diagnose and assess the progression of retinopathy where retinal changes occur. Retinopathy could be brought about by hypertension or diabetes.

A2　C

A stethoscope may be used for auscultation of heart sounds or breath sounds. Abnormal breath sounds such as wheezes and bronchial breath sounds may occur with airways obstruction or respiratory tract infections.

A3　E

A reflex hammer is used to evaluate deep tendon reflexes. It is used to assess damage to the spinal reflex arc such as after a cerebrovascular accident.

Questions 4–6

An understanding of the control of hormones and mechanisms that affect their production and release is essential to understand the pathology of the disease states that are related to the endocrine system.

A4   E

Human chorionic gonadotrophin is a hormone that is secreted by trophoblastic cells in the placenta and is excreted in the urine of pregnant women. It stimulates the corpus luteum to secrete oestrogen and progesterone and to decrease lymphocyte activation. Its presence in urine is used as the indicator for pregnancy in pregnancy tests.

A5   B

C peptide is an inactive residue of insulin formation in the beta cells of the pancreas. It is degraded in the kidney. Measurement of serum C peptide may be used in diabetic patients who are being treated with insulin and who have anti-insulin antibodies. Diminished kidney function may lead to increased amounts of C peptide in serum.

A6   D

Prolactin is a hormone that is produced by the anterior pituitary gland. In conjunction with other hormones such as oestrogen and progesterone, it stimulates development of mammary glands. After parturition, it stimulates and maintains breast milk production. Prolactin blood levels are used in the diagnosis of prolactin-secreting pituitary adenomas.

Questions 7–26

A7   A

Creatine kinase (CK) is an enzyme that is found in heart muscle, skeletal muscle and the brain. There are three isoenzymes: CK-BB (CPK1) which is predominantly found in the brain and lungs, CK-MB (CPK2) mainly found in myocardial cells and CK-MM (CPK3) which consists of circulatory CK. Creatine kinase blood levels rise when these muscle or nerve cells are injured.

Differential elevations of the three isoenzymes indicate the type of tissue that has been damaged. A rise in CK-BB occurs after a cerebrovascular accident or pulmonary infarction. CK-MB is elevated after a myocardial infarction and in unstable angina. However, severe skeletal muscle injury may also elevate CK-MB. CK-MM levels are increased in myopathies, after vigorous exercise or surgery.

A8   D

Auscultation of bowel sounds is undertaken to identify bowel obstruction or ileus. Ileus is a condition where there is an obstruction of the intestines resulting from immobility or mechanical obstruction. Ileus may be due to opioid drugs and could occur postoperatively because of the administration of opioid drugs and anaesthesia. After a surgical intervention, bowel sounds are monitored using a stethoscope to eliminate ileus. Normal bowel sounds indicate peristalsis and may be audible without the use of a stethoscope.

A9   B

A complete blood count (CBC) is a series of tests on a blood sample to present red blood cell count, haemoglobin level, haematocrit, red blood cell indices (mean corpuscular volume, mean corpuscular haemoglobin, mean corpuscular concentration), white blood cell count and differential count for different components, blood smear and platelet count.

A10   B

The erythrocyte sedimentation rate (ESR) is a non-specific test that indicates conditions of inflammation, infection, malignancy and tissue necrosis or infarction. The test is a measure of the rate at which red blood cells settle out of mixed venous blood over a specified period. The test requires that a blood sample is aspirated into a calibrated sedimentation tube and blood is allowed to settle usually for 60 minutes. ESR together with other indicators may be used to evaluate disease progression.

A11   A

Gastro-oesophageal reflux disease (GORD) is usually due to reflux oesophagitis, which results in acid regurgitation. Stomach contents which have a low pH are refluxed into the oesophagus and the oesophageal mucosa has very little, if any, protection against acidic contents. Dysphagia, which is difficulty in swallowing, may sometimes occur in GORD. Stricture formation of the oesophagus may take place in GORD, owing to the inflammation caused by acid regurgitation.

A12   C

A mixture of magnesium hydroxide and aluminium salts in antacid preparations is referred to as co-magaldrox. Antacid preparations are used for the symptomatic management of dyspepsia, gastro-oesophageal reflux and gastric pain. Patients are advised to use the preparation after meals and at bedtime when required. Co-magaldrox preparations have the advantage that they eliminate the side-effects of magnesium salts (diarrhoea) and aluminium salts (constipation) as they cancel each other out. Patients should be advised not to take antacid preparations at the same time as other medications as antacids may impair absorption of the other drugs. Antacids may damage enteric-coated tablets, resulting in the dissolution of the drug in the stomach, thus defeating the purpose of using an enteric-coated formulation.

A13   E

Some drugs may cause phototoxic or photoallergic reactions if the patient is exposed to ultraviolet light. When patients taking amiodarone (for arrhythmias) are exposed to direct sunlight or to sun lamps, photosensitivity may occur owing to a phototoxic reaction. A skin reaction may occur and this may continue for some weeks after treatment when amiodarone is stopped. Patients using amiodarone should be advised to use total sunblock preparations, to wear protective clothing and to avoid exposure to sun.

A14   A

Immunoglobulins are used in clinical practice to induce passive immunity and therefore to present immediate protection against an infectious disease. Human immunoglobulins may be of two types: normal immunoglobulin or specific immunoglobulins. Normal immunoglobulin presents antibodies against several infectious diseases, whereas specific immunoglobulins present a specific antibody such as hepatitis B immunoglobulin. Human immunoglobulins are prepared from pooled plasma or serum of human donors. The human donor material is tested for presence of hepatitis B surface antigen and for antibodies against hepatitis C virus and human immunodeficiency virus. Human immunoglobulins are preferred to antisera (immunoglobulins) as they are associated with a lower incidence of hypersensitivity reactions.

A15   B

Glue ear, also referred to as sero-mucinous otitis media, is a condition where there is an accumulation of viscous mucous fluid in the middle ear, usually occurring after repeated attacks of acute otitis media. It occurs most commonly in children. Glue ear may also be found in association with inflammation of the sinuses and blockage of the eustachian tube. Deafness or difficulty in hearing is usually the presenting symptom and in some cases this may go unnoticed and lead to permanent hearing loss.

A16   B

Hepatitis C is a viral infection that is transmitted through contact with contaminated blood such as when sharing needles and through intravenous drug misuse or the transfusion of infected blood. In hepatitis C, the aim of treatment is to achieve the clearance of the virus, which is sustained for at least 6 months after treatment has stopped. This reduces the risk of cirrhosis and hepatocellular carcinoma. Patients may require a liver transplant to prevent death caused by cirrhosis. Interferon alfa is used in combination with ribavirin (antiviral drug). Peginterferon alfa consists of a polyethylene glycol-conjugated derivative of interferon alfa. Pegylation results in increasing the availability of interferon in blood and therefore halflife is extended so that the dosing frequency that is required is reduced.

A17   A

A stroke, also referred to as a cerebrovascular accident, is due to acute neurological dysfunction of vascular origin in focal areas of the brain. It may present as a completed stroke, where the signs and symptoms occur for more than 24 h, or a transient ischaemic attack if the signs disappear within a few minutes or at most within 24 h. Patients with transient ischaemic attacks or stroke are at an increased risk of further stroke, myocardial infarction or sudden death. Pharmacotherapy that could be used to prevent these sequalae include long-term prophylaxis with daily aspirin. An angiotensin-converting enzyme (ACE) inhibitor should be considered, especially in patients with hypertension, to reduce blood pressure and for the prophylaxis of cardiovascular events. Hypercholesterolaemia is a risk factor for atherosclerosis and cardiovascular disease. Statins may be considered to decrease plasma-cholesterol concentrations.

A18   B

Colorectal cancers may be classified according to the Duke's classification, which was originally described in 1932, or according to the TNM classification. A stage III or a Duke's C tumour implies that tumour cells have invaded the musculature and that there is lymph node involvement. There is a 10–40% chance of a 5-year survival rate. Patients with stage III colorectal cancer should receive adjuvant chemotherapy to decrease the high risk of recurrence. Choice of adjuvant chemotherapy is based on a risk-to-benefit ratio for the individual patient who is usually asymptomatic after tumour resection. Side-effects and the method of administration should be taken into account when deciding which drugs to use. Drugs that do not require an invasive administration, such as drugs presented in oral formulations – for example, capecitabine – are preferred to drugs that require lengthy intravenous infusions such as irinotecan.

A19 B

Calcium supplementation increases net calcium absorption and decreases bone turnover. Many adults are in negative calcium balance throughout their lives, an imbalance that worsens with age and increases the risk of osteoporosis and bone fracture. Calcium supplementation presents calcium salts as tablets, chewable tablets or effervescent tablets. The patient is required to take a sustained daily intake of the calcium supplement for a prolonged time. Poor compliance is quite common with individuals stopping intake or taking the supplementation intermittently. Products containing calcium and vitamin D may be used in the management of osteoporosis to prevent fractures. Cacitriol, a metabolite of vitamin D, enhances the absorption of calcium from the small intestine. Different calcium salts may be used for supplementation such as calcium lactate, calcium carbonate and calcium gluconate. Calcium carbonate has the highest calcium content per gram of salt.

A20 C

Myopia is an ophthalmic condition resulting in parallel rays being focused in front of the retina. It may be caused by an elongation of the eyeball or by an error of refraction. The condition is also called nearsightedness or shortsightedness as affected individuals cannot clearly see objects that are more than a metre from the eye. Concave lenses for spectacles or contact lenses are used to correct the error.

A21 B

Patients following a low-fat diet should be advised to increase fibre intake which is found in fruits, green leafy vegetables, root vegetables, cereals and breads. This will increase satiety and may interfere with fat absorption due to adsorption with fat molecules. Saturated fat is found mainly in food of animal origin such as beef, pork, lamb and whole-milk products. A diet high in saturated fats results in high serum cholesterol levels and high serum low-density lipoprotein cholesterol levels. Polyunsaturated fat is predominantly present in fish, corn, sunflower seeds, soybeans and walnuts. Patients following a low-fat diet should restrict their intake of saturated fats and concentrate more on polyunsaturated fat.

A22   C

Atopic eczema is a skin condition characterised by pruritus and inflammation. A prominent feature is dry skin. Atopic eczema may become infected because of the patient scratching the area, which is intensely pruritic. The skin is more susceptible to microbial colonisation because of dehydration and inflammation. Patients should be advised to avoid scratching the area and to use emollients and emollient bath oils instead of regular soap and bubble baths when bathing. These can be used and applied as needed.

A23   D

Phenytoin is an antiepileptic drug that has a narrow therapeutic drug index. Monitoring of plasma concentrations is used to reduce phenytoin toxicity by assessing that the plasma concentration is within the therapeutic range. It is particularly useful when patient is started on the treatment, during dose adjustments to achieve seizure control or when the patient complains of side-effects that may be attributed to high plasma concentrations of phenytoin. In cancer chemotherapy, side-effects, particularly neutropenia and other specific side-effects such as cardiac toxicity for doxorubicin, are the dose-limiting parameters that are used. Alteplase is a fibrinolytic drug that is used as quickly as possible in myocardial infarction, stroke and pulmonary embolism. Alteplase is a glycosylated protein and it is cleared rapidly from plasma mainly by metabolism in the liver.

A24   B

Irritable bowel syndrome is a condition where patients complain of diarrhoea or constipation, abdominal pain and bloating. The condition may impact negatively on the patient's social life as they may feel that their symptoms restrict their activities. The condition may be associated with stress and depression.

A25   A

Kidney transplantation is necessary when there is irreversible failure of the kidney. There are a number of complications associated with this intervention, including donor identification, organ preservation and organ rejection. Immunosuppressive agents are used to promote acceptance of the donor organ, while maintaining as much as possible a functional immune system. Azathioprine, prednisolone, which is a corticosteroid, and ciclosporin are used in kidney transplantation to prevent organ rejection.

A26   B

Anaemia in cancer patients may be chemotherapy-induced or may be due to the tumour. The tumour may result in bone marrow infiltration or lead to gastrointestinal blood loss. The process of development of anaemia in cancer patients may not be clearly understood. Anaemia develops insidiously. It may be corrected with the use of human recombinant erythropoietin, particularly if it is chemotherapy-induced. Erythropoietin and darbepoetin, which is the hyperglycosylated derivative of erythropoietin, are used to correct anaemia.

Questions 27–34

On admission, LJ is taking bendroflumethiazide (thiazide diuretic), warfarin (anticoagulant) and potassium chloride supplements to counteract potassium loss brought about by the thiazide diuretic. She has a past history of hypertension and asthma and she is admitted with atrial fibrillation. Atrial fibrillations are cardiac arrhythmias characterised by disorganised electrical activity in the atria. Clinical symptoms include shortness of breath, irregular pulse, dizziness, acute syncopal episodes and heart failure symptoms. Treatment goals are restoration of sinus rhythm and prevention of further recurrences. On admission she is started on digoxin (cardiac glycoside) and perindopril (angiotensin-converting enzyme inhibitor).

A27 B

Atrial fibrillation is a supraventricular arrhythmia that may be precipitated by cardiovascular disease that causes atrial distension, such as hypertension, ischaemia and infarction. It represents a chaotic, disorganised atrial activation. Ventricular premature beats constitute a form of ventricular arrhythmias.

A28 B

An electrocardiogram may be undertaken for LJ to confirm the nature of the arrhythmias, and 24-h recordings may be preferred to allow monitoring. Drugs such as amitriptyline (tricyclic antidepressant) and lithium (antimanic drug) may interfere with the QT interval which represents the time between depolarisation and repolarisation of the ventricles. Selective serotonin re-uptake inhibitors such as fluoxetine are not associated with prolonged QT intervals.

A29 B

Occurrence of atrial fibrillation increases the risk of stroke and heart failure.

A30 B

In atrial fibrillation, the ventricular response results in a rapid ventricular rate. Digoxin is a cardiac glycoside that may be used in the management of atrial fibrillation to control ventricular response. Beta-blockers are used to control the ventricular rate. They should be avoided in LJ as she has a past history of asthma. Beta-blockers should be used with caution in asthma as they may cause bronchospasms. Digoxin increases the force of myocardial contraction and decreases conductivity in the atrioventricular node. It does not interfere with blood pressure.

A31   A

Digoxin has a narrow therapeutic range but plasma concentration is not the only factor indicating risk of toxicity. There is inter-individual variability in the sensitivity of the conducting system or the myocardium to digoxin. Lower doses should be started in elderly patients and the drug should be used with care as a decreased renal elimination may result in toxic effects. Digoxin should also be used with care in renal impairment and in patients who recently have had an infarction. In renal impairment, the electrolyte disturbances associated with renal disease such as hypokalaemia predispose to toxicity. Caution should be employed with its use following a myocardial infarction because of increased sensitivity of the myocardium.

A32   A

When LJ is hospitalised, serum potassium levels should be checked and monitored to avoid occurrence of hypokalaemia. In LJ hypokalaemia may precipitate further arrhythmias, and increases the risk of digoxin toxicity. Plasma digoxin concentration is useful to ensure that the dose results in a plasma concentration that is within the therapeutic range and therefore the risk of toxicity is minimised. The ventricular rate at rest should be monitored to assess outcomes of therapy and to assess ventricular response to atrial fibrillation.

A33   D

LJ is started on perindopril because she has uncontrolled blood pressure. Angiotensin-converting enzyme (ACE) inhibitors are preferred to beta-blockers in patients with asthma. For the management of hypertension, the recommended initial dose is 4 mg daily. LJ was started on a lower dose because she is an elderly patient and she is receiving bendroflumethiazide, which is a diuretic. LJ is more at risk of developing first-dose hypotension. The dose is given at night to limit injuries associated with hypotension.

A34   D

ACE inhibitors such as perindopril cause potassium retention because they inhibit secretion of aldosterone. They should not be used concurrently with potassium supplements and potassium-sparing diuretics as there is a risk of the development of hyperkalaemia, which should be avoided particularly in LJ as it poses a risk of cardiac rhythm disturbances, namely ventricular fibrillation and cardiac asystole. Perindopril should be continued for the management of hypertension. Sustained hypertension in LJ may have precipitated atrial fibrillation and may precipitate other cardiovascular conditions. Warfarin therapy should be continued as patients with chronic atrial fibrillation are at risk of developing embolism that may lead to stroke and death. In LJ the use of aspirin is not indicated as it may precipitate an asthmatic attack.

Questions 35–43

AX presents with symptoms of rheumatoid arthritis flare-up. On admission, AX is receiving methotrexate as a disease-modifying antirheumatic drug, fluvastatin (statin), folic acid and paracetamol as required. Clinical laboratory investigations are normal except for a slight depression in the red blood cell count. Further investigations are required before a cause of anaemia can be established. The red blood cell count may be repeated and haemoglobin levels measured. AX has a previous history of peptic ulceration and colonic polyps in addition to rheumatoid arthritis. AX is administered methylprednisolone for one day.

A35   D

Rheumatoid arthritis is a progressive disease that is associated with deterioration in patient mobility and a reduction in life expectancy of 7 years in males and 3 years in women. The aims of treatment in rheumatoid arthritis are to relieve pain, inflammation and symptoms of flare-ups, to prevent joint destruction and to preserve functional ability so that the patient can lead as normal a lifestyle as possible.

A36   A

Monitoring of outcomes of therapy and of disease progression includes biochemical tests where changes in inflammatory markers are followed. Biochemical tests that are undertaken include the measurement of C-reactive protein (CRP), erythrocyte sedimentation rate (ESR), rheumatoid factor and antinuclear antibodies. These markers are not specific to rheumatoid disease and so changes in levels may be experienced when patient has an inflammatory condition.

A37   B

In AX, methylprednisolone is administered by slow intravenous infusion as a single dose to control symptoms associated with the flare-up and to induce remission. It has glucocorticoid effects resulting in an anti-inflammatory action due to suppression of cytokines. Administration, especially parenteral, results in a rapid improvement in symptoms. It is used only to reduce symptoms of flare-up and should not be continued orally in the long term.

A38   D

Corticosteroids are associated with the development of peptic ulceration. Use of corticosteroids in AX should be undertaken with caution and considered only to treat aggressive flare-ups or until the condition is managed with different disease-modifying antirheumatic agents. There are no interactions reported when methylprednisolone is used in patients receiving fluvastatin and no correlation with allergy to leflunomide.

A39   B

Methylprednisolone is a steroid with a greater glucocorticoid activity compared with prednisolone and lower mineralcorticoid effects. About 4 mg of methylprednisolone are equivalent to the anti-inflammatory activity experienced with 5 mg prednisolone. Methylprednisolone is similar to other corticosteroids and is rapidly absorbed from the gastrointestinal tract when administered orally.

A40   E

In addition to anti-inflammatory and immunosuppressive effects, glucocorticoid activity results in metabolic effects including a decrease in peripheral glucose utilisation and an increase in gluconeogenesis. This may lead to hyperglycaemia and increased insulin requirements in diabetic patients. When measuring blood glucose, consideration has to be given to whether the measurement was undertaken post-prandially or when the patient was fasting.

A41   B

Cytokine inhibitors such as infliximab, etanercept, adalimumab are used as disease-modifying antirheumatic drugs in the management of rheumatoid arthritis. They may be considered to be additional treatment with methotrexate if the frequency of flare-ups increases in AX.

A42   A

Methotrexate is commonly prescribed as a weekly dose. Dispensing errors and errors in drug administration, where the patient takes the drug on a daily basis may occur. Patient should be counselled to ensure understanding of the dosage regimen. Nausea and vomiting may occur with drug administration. Bone marrow suppression is another side-effect of methotrexate. Patients should be advised to report any signs of infection and a full blood count should be performed every few months.

A43   E

AX is prescribed folic acid to be taken weekly to prevent the stomatitis that may occur as a result of methotrexate therapy. Folic acid is used to counter-act the folate-antagonist action of methotrexate. Folic acid is reduced in the body to tetrahydrofolate.

Questions 44–47

MB is complaining of palpitations, where the patient is aware of his or her's heart beat, and this may present as a distressing phenomenon. Palpitations may be signs of arrhythmias and tachycardia.

A44   B

Moxonidine is a centrally acting drug that blocks imidazoline and alpha$_2$-adrenoceptors. It is used for the treatment of mild-to-moderate hypertension, especially where the condition is unresponsive to first-line therapy.

A45   D

Methyldopa and clonidine are two other antihypertensive drugs that are centrally acting. Moxonidine is a newer drug that is associated with fewer side-effects owing to its central action. Doxazosin blocks the alpha-adrenocep-tors in the blood vessel walls and therefore brings about vasodilation. In hyper-tension doxazosin and other alpha-adrenoceptor blocking drugs are used in conjunction with other antihypertensives. Alpha-adrenoceptor blockers are used as single therapy in the management of benign prostatic hyperplasia.

Hydralazine is a vasodilator that is used as an adjunct to other antihypertensives in the management of moderate-to-severe hypertension.

A46   E

Moxonidine is structurally similar to clonidine. As for clonidine, abrupt withdrawal should be avoided as it may be associated with an increased cathecolamine release that may be manifested with agitation, sweating, tachycardia, headache, nausea and rebound hypertension. MB may be presenting with symptoms of palpitations caused by this effect as there are no other indications of symptoms related to heart failure and stroke. Bradycardia, severe arrhythmias, severe heart failure, severe ischaemic heart disease and severe renal or hepatic impairment should be excluded before moxonidine therapy is started again.

A47   C

Long-standing hypertension may cause complications associated with cardiovascular dysfunction, such as myocardial infarction, stroke and peripheral vascular disease in the retina, kidneys and extremities. Hypertensive patients should undergo tests to assess the presence or extent of end organ damage. Tests include retinal examination, electrocardiogram, chest radiograph, kidney function tests.

Questions 48–52

RB has systemic sclerosis, which is a type of scleroderma where there is chronic hardening and thickening of the skin caused by collagen formation. Raynaud's phenomenon is often a concomitant condition. Raynaud's phenomenon is characterised by intermittent attacks of ischaemia in the extremities of the body especially fingers and toes. On admission RB was taking pentoxifylline (vasodilator) and nifedipine (calcium-channel blocker).

A48 E

During an attack of Raynaud's disease, finger discoloration is common. Pain is not usually a prominent symptom. RB is presenting with swelling, tenderness and mild erythema. There is also a clear discharge beneath the nail fold which may indicate infection. The management plan should include use of an anti-bacterial agent to treat the infection that may have precipitated the symptoms. Co-amoxiclav given as an intravenous therapy is an appropriate first choice anti-bacterial agent as it is a broad spectrum agent. Co-amoxiclav consists of clavulanic acid potentiated amoxicillin.

A49 B

Pentoxifylline is a xanthine derivative that has vasodilating properties. It increases blood flow to ischaemic tissues and results in an improvement of tissue oxygenation in the affected areas. Side-effects of pentoxifylline include gastrointestinal disturbances, dizziness, agitation, sleep disturbances and headache. Hypotension may also occur and pentoxifylline should be used with caution in patients with hypotension. Pentoxifylline may be used as long-term therapy in the management of Raynaud's disease to reduce severe symptoms and the frequency of acute attacks.

A50 B

Factors that reduce blood flow in the fingers increase the risk of an acute attack. RB should be advised to avoid exposure to cold temperatures and to use lined gloves when handling food in freezers. She should use gloves in winter to protect them from the cold. She should be advised to stop smoking and information on smoking cessation should be provided. Emotional stress and anxiety may also precipitate an attack.

A51   D

Atenolol is a beta-adrenoceptor blocking drug. These drugs result in a reduced peripheral circulation leading to coldness of extremities and may exacerbate an acute attack of Raynaud's disease.

A52   E

Nifedipine is a calcium-channel blocker which, unlike verapamil, has more influence on the peripheral and coronary vessels than on the myocardium. Nifedipine is a vasodilator that reduces the frequency and severity of vasospastic effects in Raynaud's phenomenon. Its effect is better when started early during the disease process. The use of a modified-release formulation reduces variations in blood pressure and decreases reflex tachycardia. Patient should be advised to swallow the tablet whole.

Questions 53–59

FG is admitted with symptoms of pulmonary oedema, chest infection and angina. Her clinical laboratory tests, indicate hypokalaemia and leucocytosis. She also has a high creatine kinase value which, together with the ST depression and T wave flattening, indicate recent ischaemia. Cardiomegaly is brought about by congestive heart failure. FG's blood glucose level is extremely high. On admission FG's drug therapy consisted of paroxetine (selective serotonin re-uptake inhibitor), potassium chloride supplement, verapamil (calcium-channel blocker), dipyridamole (antiplatelet), bumetanide (loop diuretic) and multivitamins.

A53   A

On admission aims of treatment for FG are to control blood glucose levels, to treat infection, to reduce pulmonary oedema and to provide prophylaxis against ischaemic events. After an infarct, diabetic patients present with a high blood glucose level as a result of a stress response by the body. Insulin is required to reduce high blood glucose and patient should be maintained on insulin therapy until stabilised. An assessment whether patient should continue to receive antidiabetic treatment is required. High glucose levels, together with the other disease states, increase FG's risk of ischaemic attacks which may be associated with morbidity and mortality. Nitrates such as isosorbide dinitrate are administered parenterally to prevent ischaemic attacks and to relieve patient from the ischaemic pain. Nitrates are vasodilators. They bring about an improvement in collateral blood flow in the heart and promote reperfusion, thus limiting infarct size and preserve functional tissue. The use of aspirin after an ischaemic event is associated with a lower risk of secondary thrombotic cerebrovascular and cardiovascular disease.

A54   A

FG has presented with hypokalaemia, which is corrected by increasing the dose of potassium chloride supplements. Serum potassium levels should be monitored. One of the complications of myocardial infarction is heart failure and this is particularly relevant for FG, who already has a history of heart failure. FG is presenting with symptoms of heart failure, and bumetanide therapy may be switched to intravenous therapy for a few days until the oedema is controlled. Verapamil is a calcium-channel blocker which slows conduction in the atrioventricular node. Verapamil may cause worsening of heart failure so it is recommended to stop verapamil therapy during this phase.

A55   B

Oxygen therapy is started in the emergency department so as to provide support to FG, who presents with shortness of breath. Oxygen is administered with masks delivering 35% oxygen. As it is being administered intermittently there is no need to use a nasal cannula; this is preferred when the patient is going to require long-term administration of oxygen. Administering oxygen by a nasal cannula decreases the interference caused by oxygen administration on eating, drinking and talking because the mouth is not obstructed. An oxygen concentration of 35% does not require humidification with a nebuliser during administration.

A56   E

Paroxetine is a selective serotonin reuptake inhibitor (SSRI). SSRIs together with tricyclic antidepressants (TCAs) are used in the management of depression. SSRIs and TCAs have similar efficacy but they differ in the side-effect profile. The preference to use SSRIs is based on fewer antimuscarinic and cardiotoxic side-effects. SSRIs may cause gastrointestinal effects, and side-effects include movement disorders and dyskinesias. Paroxetine is a phenylpiperidine derivative. Fluoxetine is another SSRI with similar properties to paroxetine. Fluoxetine has a different chemical structure as it is a phenylpropylamine derivative.

A57   B

Dipyridamole is a phosphodiesterase inhibitor and an adenosine reuptake inhibitor. It has antiplatelet and vasodilating properties. It is used for secondary prevention of ischaemic stroke and transient ischaemic attacks. Its use in FG should be monitored as dipyridamole should be used with caution in rapidly worsening angina. Reports of transient myocardial ischaemia in patients with unstable angina have been documented. Side-effects associated with the use of dipyridamole include nausea, vomiting, diarrhoea, dizziness, myalgia, throbbing headache, hypotension, hot flushes and tachycardia. Bleeding disorders are not a common side-effect. Increased bleeding may occur during or after surgery.

A58   A

A chest radiograph reveals cardiomegaly in FG. Cardiomegaly or enlargement of the heart, usually caused by left ventricular hypertrophy, occurs to accommodate the increased ventricular load. In heart failure, the ability of cardiac muscle to respond to an increased preload through increased elastic recoil is diminished. Sustained increased preload leads to loss of elastic recoil possibilities. The increased ventricular load associated with cardiomegaly may lead to pulmonary congestion. An increase in oxygen requirements of cardiac cells leads to development of tachycardia, arrhythmias and myocardial ischaemia.

A59   B

Bumetanide may result in water and electrolyte imbalance, which may be manifested by hypotension, muscle cramps, headache, dry mouth, thirst and weakness. Dipyridamole may also cause hypotension. If the patient is started on a nitrate, it also may cause hypotension. Blood pressure should be monitored in FG, particularly during changes in drug therapy.

Questions 60–66

AP has a history of diabetes and cardiovascular disease. She presents with chest pain and symptoms of unwellness. As she reports that pain started at rest and is occurring from time to time, AP probably has unstable angina. Stable angina is not associated with chest pain at rest. The ECG shows T wave inversion, indicating recent infarction and this is confirmed from the elevated creatine kinase level. On admission AP is taking candesartan (angiotensin-II receptor antagonist), clopidrogel (antiplatelet), isosorbide mononitrate (nitrate), fluvastatin (statin), amlodipine (calcium-channel blocker), carvedilol (beta-adrenoceptor blocker), bumetanide (loop diuretic), and isophane insulin (intermediate-acting insulin).

A60   B

Carvedilol is a non-cardioselective beta-adrenoceptor blocker. It blocks the beta-receptors of the sympathetic nervous system in the heart, peripheral vasculature, bronchi, pancreas and liver. A characteristic of carvedilol is that it also has vasodilating properties and it is used in the management of heart failure, where it has been shown to decrease mortality. Unlike atenolol, carvedilol has high lipid solubility.

A61 B

Hypotension may occur as a common side-effect of a number of drugs that are included in AP's treatment. Isosorbide mononitrate is a vasodilator that presents postural hypotension as a common side-effect. Carvedilol, which also has vasodilating properties, may also cause postural hypotension. Amlodipine and candesartan too may cause hypotension, and the risk is higher in patients who are taking diuretics and may develop dehydration. Amlodipine commonly induces flushing especially at the start of therapy and isosorbide mononitrate may also cause flushing.

A62 E

Candesartan is an ester prodrug and it is hydrolysed to the active form during absorption from the gastrointestinal tract. It is an angiotensin-II receptor antagonist that blocks the angiotensin receptors, resulting in a decreased effect of angiotensin II. Angiotensin-II receptor antagonists have similar properties to angiotensin-converting enzyme (ACE) inhibitors. Both classes of drugs are used in the management of hypertension and heart failure. An important feature of angiotensin-II receptor antagonists is that, unlike ACE inhibitors, they do not inhibit the breakdown of bradykinin. This activity, which occurs with ACE inhibitors, is associated with cough as a side-effect of ACE inhibitors. Cough does not usually occur with candesartan and other angiotensin-II receptor antagonists and in fact they may be used in patients who are intolerant to ACE inhibitors owing to this side-effect. It has a long elimination halflife (about 9 h) and is usually given as a once-daily dose. Angiotensin-II receptor antagonists should be used with caution in renal artery stenosis as they may reduce glomerular filtration rate precipitating renal failure.

A63   B

Isophane insulin is an intermediate-acting insulin preparation that allows twice-daily injection. AP should be advised to avoid episodes of hypoglycaemia by correctly following the dose administration of insulin and keeping a standard food intake pattern. The risk of hypoglycaemia is highest before meals and at night. A response to hypoglycaemia is the activation of the sympathetic nervous system and adrenal medulla. This response leads to tremor, pallor, sweating, shivering, palpitations and anxiety, which are early clinical signs of hypoglycaemia. Such a response increases oxygen demand in the cardiac muscle and may precipitate angina attacks and myocardial infarction in AP. During an anginal attack, glycaemic control is lost because of the resulting metabolic stress and insulin requirements are increased.

A64   D

Isosorbide mononitrate is a nitrate that is used in angina. Nitrates are potent coronary vasodilators and bring about a reduced venous return. It has an elimination halflife of 4–5 h. Modified-release formulations are available where dosage regimen is once daily. The advantages of a modified-release formulation is that major peaks and troughs in drug blood levels are avoided and this results in better control of anginal symptoms. Once-daily dosing of the modified-release formulation results in low blood-nitrate concentrations towards the end of the 24-h period, and this avoids the development of the tolerance associated with nitrates. Isosorbide mononitrate is metabolised to inactive metabolites such as isosorbide and isosorbide glucuronide.

A65   B

Fluvastatin is a statin that acts as a 3-hydroxyl-3-methylglutaryl coenzyme A (HMG CoA) reductase inhibitor. Statins are used as lipid regulating drugs and they reduce low-density-lipoprotein cholesterol (LDL cholesterol). AP should be advised to report muscle pain immediately as statins may cause myalgia and muscle weakness, which may be associated with myopathy, which may progress to rhabdomyolysis and renal failure. Occurrence of myopathy and rhabdomyolysis is associated with an elevated creatine kinase. Statins should be used with caution in patients with a history of liver disease and are not indicated during active liver disease. Liver function tests are required before starting statin therapy. Statins should be used with caution in severe renal impairment. Renal function tests should be carried out at baseline. AP was taking fluvastatin 80 mg at night, which is the maximum recommended dose. Hypothyroidism should be corrected before starting statins as correction may resolve the hyperlipidaemia. Thyroid function tests should be carried out, especially in elderly patients who may have a hypothyroid state with sub-clinical symptoms. Simvastatin is another statin that may be used as an alternative and the maximum therapeutic dose is 80 mg daily.

A66   A

Unstable angina may present with negative outcomes and requires immediate hospitalisation. Complete bed rest is recommended for a few days. AP should be started on oxygen, isosorbide mononitrate is changed to a nitrate intravenous infusion, such as isosorbide dinitrate injections. AP is already on clopidrogel which is an expensive antiplatelet drug. Clopidrogel is used in the management of unstable angina. Heparin or the low-molecular-weight (LMWH) heparins may be used for the first 2–5 days. Use of heparin products with clopidrogel increases risk of bleeding.

Questions 67–70

KB presents with symptoms associated with disorders of the urinary tract. She is complaining of dysuria (painful urination) that occurs as a result of infection or obstruction in the urinary tract. KB also presents with urinary urgency and urinary frequency.

A67 B

The symptoms presented by KB are suggestive of a lower urinary tract infection also known as cystitis, where the bladder and urethra are involved. Bacteria may ascend the urinary tract to affect the kidneys leading to acute pyelonephritis. A common causative organism of cystitis and acute pyelonephritis is *Escherichia coli*. Vulvovaginitis is an inflammation of the vulva and vagina, which is not associated with urinary urgency and urinary frequency.

A68 B

Patient should be asked about occurrence of fever. This helps to differentiate between cystitis and acute pyelonephritis. The latter is associated with fever, chills, pain in the sides and nausea, in addition to the urinary symptoms. Pharmacists can carry out a urinalysis to confirm diagnosis. Bacterial urinary tract infection leads to an alkaline urine pH as a number of organisms, including *E. coli*, are urea-splitting organisms. Haematuria and the presence of nitrites in urine caused by bacterial enzymes that reduce urinary nitrates to nitrites also occur. The test may be repeated after the recommended treatment has been completed so as to confirm that bacterial infection has been eradicated. Culturing of bacteria present in urine from mid-stream samples may be required to identify causative organism, to use anti-bacterial agents that are active against the particular microorganism. However, in the normal setting, when the patient is presenting with primary symptoms and there are no other complications, this test may be delayed.

A69 B

KB is advised to drink lots of water to flush out the urinary system and dilute the microorganisms. Alkalinisation of urine may be used to relieve the discomfort caused by the urinary tract infection. Potassium citrate salts are used. If KB has signs of acute pyelonephritis or symptoms have not subsided with potassium citrate salts, then antibacterial agents are required.

A70   B

Antibacterial agents that are active against *E. coli* are recommended for the management of cystitis and acute pyelonephritis. Drugs used include broad-spectrum penicillins such as amoxicillin and co-amoxiclav, broad-spectrum cephalosporins such as cefalexin and cefuroxime, trimethoprim and quinolones such as ciprofloxacin.

Questions 71–75

SC is presenting with high blood pressure during the first month of pregnancy. Increased blood pressure during pregnancy may be associated with pre-eclampsia and intrauterine growth retardation.

A71   B

As there is hypertension before the first 20–24 weeks of pregnancy, there is a probability that hypertension was pre-existing before conception. SC has a higher risk of developing pre-eclampsia. Pre-eclampsia presents with hypertension, proteinuria and oedema. Complications of pre-eclampsia include early delivery, low-birth-weight and eclampsia, which can result in maternal and fetal death. Eclampsia is associated with seizures and coma. Hypertension may be due to secondary causes. However, this cannot be deduced from the clinical presentation.

A72   A

During pregnancy, SC should be monitored to assess the development of the symptoms of pre-eclampsia, namely hypertension, proteinuria and changes in fetal growth. During check-ups SC should have her blood pressure measured and urinalysis routinely carried out. Fetal growth should be regularly monitored.

A73   A

During pregnancy, the use of thiazide diuretics, beta-adrenoceptor blockers, angiotensin-converting enzyme (ACE) inhibitors and angiotensin-II receptor inhibitors should be avoided. Thiazide diuretics may cause neonatal thrombo-cytopenia. ACE inhibitors and angiotensin-II receptor inhibitors may affect maternal renal function and lead to intrauterine death. Beta-blockers may cause intrauterine growth retardation. They may be used after the third trimester if other drugs are not effective or are contraindicated.

A74   E

Methyldopa, a centrally acting antihypertensive agent, may be used in pregnancy. It has a very good safety record when used for the management of hypertension in pregnancy. Hydralazine, a vasodilator, may be used after the third trimester.

A75   B

Labetalol is a non-cardioselective drug that acts as a competitive antagonist to alpha and beta-receptors in the sympathetic nervous system. Owing to its action on the alpha receptors, it results in vasodilation leading to a lower peripheral resistance. The chemical structure of labetalol has two optical centres and formulations available clinically may present a mixture of the four diasteriomers.

Questions 76–80

HG is presenting with symptoms of allergic rhinitis. Allergy results from an inappropriate immune response by the body to an allergen. HG states that she has been using oxymetazoline spray, which is a direct-acting sympatho-mimetic agent that is used as a nasal decongestant.

A76   B

HG may have the perennial type of allergic rhinitis as she states that she has recurrent attacks of nasal allergy indicating that the attacks may not be seasonal. Allergens include house dust, pollen and pet fur. Exposure to the allergen(s) results in mast cells and T lymphocyte activation that lead to the release of histamine, leukotrienes, prostaglandins and kinins. Symptoms of allergic rhinitis include nasal itching, rhinorrhoea, itchy throat, sneezing and dry cough, particularly at night. Conjunctival symptoms may also occur.

A77   B

In HG, oxymetazoline provides relief against nasal congestion. Oxymetazoline is an alpha-adrenoceptor agonist and its topical administration causes nasal vasoconstriction, thus reducing swelling and congestion in the nasal mucous membranes. However, prolonged use may lead to rebound congestion, also known as rhinitis medicamentosa. Patients should be advised not to use it for more than 1 week. HG should be advised to stop using oxymetazoline. Oxymetazoline is available for topical nasal application as nasal spray or nasal drops.

A78   D

Desloratidine is an antihistamine that may be used for symptomatic relief in HG. The product may be used on a long-term basis and the non-sedating property of desloratidine is an advantage with regards to the lower incidence of sedation compared with older sedating agents. Desloratidine is an active metabolite of loratidine and it is available for oral administration on a once-daily regimen. Antihistamines reduce secretions, nasal itching, sneezing and ocular symptoms and are considered to be a first-line option in the management of mild or intermittent allergic rhinitis.

A79   E

Budesonide is a corticosteroid that was developed for inhalation for the management of asthma. It is also available as a nasal spray for use in allergic rhinitis and as an oral formulation that is used in the management of Crohn's disease. Corticosteroids are used in the treatment and prophylaxis of allergic rhinitis and asthma. Corticosteroids decrease production of cytokines and chemokines associated with the inflammatory reaction brought about after exposure to allergens.

A80   B

HG should be advised to avoid exposure to allergens. She should be advised to avoid walking in gardens and to use products to eradicate house dust mites regularly in the house. Blood in sputum (haemoptysis) is not associated with allergies or asthma but may indicate conditions such as lung cancer or infectious diseases, for example, tuberculosis. Its occurrence requires referral for assessment.

Bibliography

Armour D, Cairns C (2002). *Medicines in the Elderly,* London: Pharmaceutical Press.

Boh L E, Young L Y (2001). *Pharmacy Practice Manual: a guide to the clinical experience*, 2nd edn. Maryland: Lippincott Williams & Wilkins.

Brunton L L, Lazo S J, Parker K L, eds (2006). *Goodman & Gilman's The Pharmacological Basis of Therapeutics*, 11th edn. New York: McGraw-Hill.

Como D N (1998). *Mosby's Medical, Nursing and Allied Health Dictionary*, 5th edn. St Louis, Missouri: Mosby.

Ferguson N (2004). *Osteoporosis in Focus,* London: Pharmaceutical Press.

Grahame-Smith D G, Aronson J K (1995). *Oxford Textbook of Clinical Pharmacology and Drug Therapy*, 2nd ed. Oxford: Oxford University Press.

Greene R J, Harris N D (2000). *Pathology and Therapeutics for Pharmacists: a basis for clinical pharmacy practice,* 2nd edn. London: Pharmaceutical Press.

Mehta D K, ed. (2007). *British National Formulary,* 53rd edn. London: Pharmaceutical Press.

Pagana K D, Pagana T J (1998). *Mosby's Manual of Diagnostic and Laboratory Tests,* St Louis, Missouri: Mosby.

Patel A (2003). *Diabetes in Focus*, 2nd edn. London: Pharmaceutical Press.

Randall M D, Neil K E (2004). *Disease Management*, London: Pharmaceutical Press.

Shankie S (2001). *Hypertension in Focus*, London: Pharmaceutical Press.

Sweetman S C, ed. (2007). *Martindale: the complete drug reference,* 35th edn. London: Pharmaceutical Press.

Tietze K J (2004). *Clinical Skills for Pharmacists: a patient-focused approach*, 2nd edn. Missouri: Mosby.

Walker R, Edwards C (2003). *Clinical Pharmacy and Therapeutics*, 3rd edn. Edinburgh: Churchill Livingstone.

Appendix A

Definitions of conditions and terminology

Acne: skin condition occurring in areas where sebaceous glands are numerous presenting with comedones, papules, and pustules

Adenoma: a tumour of glandular epithelium where the cells are arranged in a characteristic glandular structure

Agranulocytosis: reduction in the number of white blood cells

Akathisia: restlessness and inability to sit still

Allergic rhinitis: a condition where nasal passages are inflamed and watery nasal discharge occurs

Anaemia: a condition where haemoglobin in blood is decreased

Anaphylaxis: hypersensitivity reaction to a previously encountered antigen that may be life-threatening

Angina: occurrence of thoracic pain associated with myocardial anoxia

Anovulatory infertility: infertility caused by failure of ovaries to produce mature ova or to release ova

Arrhythmia: deviation from normal heart beat pattern

Asthma: a respiratory condition characterised by dyspnoea and wheezing caused by bronchoconstriction and viscous bronchial secretions

Ataxia: a condition characterised by an inability to coordinate movement

Atherosclerosis: plaques consisting of cholesterol, lipids and cellular debris in the inner layers of the walls of arteries

Atopic eczema: a skin condition that is associated with intense pruritus and inflammation

Atrial fibrillation: cardiac arrhythmias caused by disorganized electrical activity in the atria

Biliary colic: pain caused by stones passing through bile ducts

Bradycardia: a decreased heart rate

Bradykinesia: general slowness of movement

Breath sounds: detection using a stethoscope of the sound of air going through the airways into the lungs

Candidiasis: infection caused by *Candida* species

Cardiac arrest: cessation of cardiac output

Cardiomegaly: enlargement of the heart

Cardiomyopathy: a condition that interferes with the structure and function of the heart

Cataract: loss of transparency of the lens of the eye

Cellulitis: an acute infection of the skin and subcutaneous tissue

Cerebrovascular accident: occlusion by an embolus in the brain or cerebrovascular haemorrhage

Cholangitis: inflammation of the bile ducts

Cholecystitis: inflammation of the gall bladder

Chronic myelocytic leukaemia: malignant neoplasia of blood-forming tissues characterised by proliferation of granular leukocytes

Chronic obstructive pulmonary disease: a respiratory condition where inspiratory and expiratory capacity of the lungs are decreased

Cirrhosis: chronic degenerative disease of the liver

Colonoscopy: diagnostic procedure to examine the colon and terminal ileum

Congestive heart failure: a condition associated with impaired pumping action of the heart

Crossmatching of blood: matching compatibility of a donor's blood with that of the recipient

Cushing's disease: a disorder where there is an increased secretion of adrenocortical steroids

Cyanosis: bluish discoloration of the skin usually in the peripheries

Cystitis: lower urinary tract infection

Deep vein thrombosis: occurrence of a thrombus in a vein

Depression: a mood disturbance disorder characterised by sadness, despair and discouragement

Diabetes: a metabolic disorder associated with a deficiency or complete lack of insulin secretion or with defects in insulin receptors

Diabetic ketoacidosis: acidosis caused by accumulation of ketones in the body resulting from extensive breakdown of fat

Diaphoresis: sweating

Dysentry: a condition caused by inflammation of the intestine caused by microorganisms or chemical irritants

Dyskinesia: impaired voluntary movement

Dysphagia: difficulty in swallowing

Dysphasia: impairment of the language aspect of speech

Dyspnoea: uncomfortable breathing

Dysuria: painful urination that occurs as a result of infection or obstruction in the urinary tract

Eclampsia: pregnancy-induced hypertension characterised by grand mal seizures, proteinuria and oedema

Encephalopathy: abnormality in the structure or function of the brain

Endocarditis: abnormality affecting the endocardium and heart valves

Erythema: redness of the skin or mucous membrane caused by dilation and congestion of superficial capillaries

Finger clubbing: enlargement of the distal phalanges of digits, most commonly of the fingers

Gastritis: a condition where there is inflammation of the lining of the stomach

Gastro-oesophageal reflux disease: a condition characterised by regurgitation of stomach contents into the oesophagus, usually caused by an incompetent lower oesophageal sphincter

Gastroscopy: visual inspection of the stomach using a gastroscope

Glaucoma: raised intraocular pressure

Gout: a condition associated with either an increased production of uric acid or a decreased excretion of uric acid

Haematemesis: vomiting of red blood indicating bleeding in the upper gastrointestinal tract

Haemophilia: condition where there is a deficiency of one of the factors required for blood coagulation

Haemoptysis: blood in sputum

Heart attack: *see Myocardial infarction*

Heart failure: *see Congestive heart failure*

Hodgkin's disease: malignant condition where there is enlargement of lymphoid tissue

Hypercalcaemia: elevated serum calcium level

Hypercholesterolaemia: increased cholesterol levels in blood

Hyperglycaemia: increased glucose level in blood

Hyperkalaemia: increased serum potassium level

Hyperlipidaemia: increased lipids in blood

Hypernatraemia: increased serum sodium level

Hyperparathyroidism: hyperactivity of the parathyroid glands resulting in excessive secretion of parathyroid hormone

Hyperplasia: an increased number of cells caused by an increased rate of cellular division

Hyperpyrexia: an extremely high body temperature

Hypersensitivity: an abnormal response of the immune system to an antigen

Hypertension: elevated blood pressure

Hyperuricaemia: an increased uric acid blood level

Hypervolaemia: increase in the intravascular fluid

Hypocalcaemia: a decreased serum calcium level

Hypochromic anaemia: a type of anaemia where there is a decreased concentration of haemoglobin in the red blood cells

Hypoglycaemia: a decreased blood glucose level

Hypokalaemia: decreased serum potassium level

Hypomagnesaemia: decreased serum magnesium level

Hypomania: a mild form of mania that is characterised by optimism

Hyponatraemia: decreased serum sodium level

Hypoprothrombinaemia: abnormally decreased amount of prothrombin in the blood

Hypotension: low blood pressure

Hypothyroidism: decreased activity of the thyroid gland

Hypoxia: inadequate oxygen supply to cells

Idiopathic thrombocytopenia purpura: a decreased amount of platelets leading to bleeding in the skin and organs

Ileus: obstruction of the intestines

Impetigo: skin infection characterised by pruritic vesicles and golden-coloured crusts

Infectious mononucleosis: a viral infection caused by the Epstein Barr virus that is characterised by fever, sore throat, swollen lymph glands, splenomegaly, and hepatomegaly

Iron deficiency anaemia: anaemia caused by supplies of iron not meeting the demand for the synthesis of haemoglobin

Irritable bowel syndrome: a condition that results in increased motility in the small and large intestines

Ischaemic heart disease: a condition that occurs in the myocardium as a result of decreased oxygen supply to myocardial tissues

Jaundice: a condition where there are increased amounts of bilirubin in the blood leading to a yellowish discoloration of the skin, mucous membranes and the eyes

Left ventricular heart failure: heart failure where the left ventricle is not contracting forcefully resulting in a depressed cardiac output and compromised peripheral perfusion

Leucoctyosis: an increase in white blood cells in the blood

Leucopenia: a decrease in white blood cells in the blood

Macroangiopathy: enlarged blood vessels

Megaloblastic anaemia: anaemia characterised by large immature dysfunctional red blood cells

Melaena: stools that contain digested blood indicating bleeding in the upper gastrointestinal tract

Metabolic acidosis: blood pH less than 7.1

Metatarsalgia: pain around the metatarsal bones

Microalbuminuria: the excretion of albumin in urine in small amounts

Microcytic anaemia: anaemia characterised by abnormally small red blood cells

Mitral stenosis: obstruction in the mitral valve which is found between the left atrium and the left ventricle in the heart

Mumps: a viral infection caused by paramyxovirus that is characterised by a swelling of the parotid glands

Muscular dystrophy: a progressive inherited condition that results in atrophy of symmetric groups of skeletal muscle

Myalgia: muscle pain

Myocardial infarction: damage to sections of cardiac muscle characterised by severe crushing chest pain

Myopathy: muscle weakness and wasting

Myopia: elongation of the eyeball leading to shortsightedness

Myositis: inflammation of muscle tissue

Necrosis: tissue death as a result of disease or injury

Neuralgia: occurs with conditions affecting the nervous system and presents with severe pain

Neuropathy: inflammation or degeneration of the peripheral nerves

Non-Hodgkin's lymphoma: malignant tumours of lymphoid tissues

Nosocomial infection: hospital-acquired infection

Oedema: accumulation of fluid in interstitial body cavities

Oesophagitis: inflammation of the oesophagus

Optic fundus: base of the interior of the eye

Orthopnoea: uncomfortable breathing; the patient needs to change posture to a particular position to breathe comfortably

Osteoarthritis: a form of arthritis where involved joints undergo degenerative changes

Osteomyelitis: infection of bone and bone marrow

Osteoporosis: a condition affecting the bone structure caused by loss of bone density

Otitis media: a condition of the middle ear caused by inflammation or infection

Paget's disease: condition associated with excessive bone destruction and abnormalities in bone repair

Pancreatitis: inflammation of the pancreas

Parkinson's disease: a degenerative neurological condition that is characterised initially by tremor at rest, pill rolling of the fingers and a shuffling gait

Petechiae: red spots on the skin as a result of small haemorrhages in the dermal or submucosal layers

Phaeochromocytoma: tumour of the chromaffin tissue of the adrenal medulla or sympathetic paraganglia

Polyuria: large quantity of urine production

Pre-eclampsia: condition during pregnancy characterised by acute hypertension after the 24th week of gestation

Prickly heat: a condition mostly caused by exposure to heat and high humidity resulting in small vesicles and papules, and erythema

Proteinuria: protein in the urine

Pruritus: itching

Pulmonary congestion: accumulation of fluid in the lungs caused by cardiovascular disease or inflammation

Pulmonary infarction: thrombus-caused obstruction in a pulmonary artery

Pulmonary oedema: accumulation of fluid in lung tissues and alveoli

Pulmonary stenosis: cardiac condition associated with hypertrophy of the right ventricle

Purpura: bleeding disorders causing haemorrhage into tissues

Pyelonephritis: infection of the kidney

Raynaud's phenomenon: a condition characterised by ischaemia of the extremities of the body, particularly the fingers

Renal artery stenosis: obstruction of the renal artery

Renal infarction: necrosis in the kidneys resulting from tissue anoxia

Retinopathy: changes in the blood vessels in the retina

Rhabdomyolysis: a condition of the skeletal muscle characterised by myoglobulinuria that may be potentially fatal

Reye's syndrome: a condition characterised by acute encephalopathy and fatty degeneration of the liver

Rheumatoid arthritis: chronic inflammatory condition characterised by symmetric inflammation of synovial joints

Rheumatoid factor: antibodies that are present in the serum of patients with rheumatoid arthritis

Sclerosis: hardening of tissues

Shingles: herpes zoster infection that presents with a unilateral rash and pain

Sjögren's syndrome: a condition that has an immunological component and is characterised by dryness of the eyes, mouth and mucous membranes

Sleep apnoea: periods during sleep of cessation of breathing of at least 10 s

Splenomegaly: enlargement of the spleen

Stomatitis: inflammation of the mouth

Stroke: cerebrovascular accident

Subdural haematoma: accumulation of blood in the subdural area

Synovitis: inflammation of the synovial membrane of a joint

Tachycardia: rapid heart rate

Tachypnoea: abnormally fast breathing rate

Tardive dyskinesia: involuntary repetitive movements of muscles in the face, limbs and trunk

Thalassaemia: a condition caused by hemolytic anaemia that occurs as a result of deficient haemoglobin synthesis

Thrombocytopenia: reduced number of platelets

Thromboembolism: blockage of a blood vessel by an embolus that is carried in the blood stream

Tinnitus: a sensation of hearing ringing sounds

Transient ischaemic attack: short episodes of cerebrovascular insufficiency caused by partial occlusion of an artery or embolism

Trigeminal neuralgia: a neurologic condition affecting the trigeminal nerve, characterised by stabbing pain occurring along the facial trigeminal nerve

Unstable angina: sudden occurrence of angina that worsens suddenly and may progress to acute myocardial infarction

Urinalysis: examination of the urine

Vulvovaginitis: inflammation of the vulva and vagina

Wilson's disease: an inherited disorder associated with a decrease in ceruloplasmin, which causes copper to accumulate slowly in the liver, and which is then released into the circulation and taken up by other tissues

Appendix B

Abbreviations and acronyms

A&E	accident and emergency
ACE	angiotensin-converting enzyme
ALP	alkaline phosphatase
ALT	alanine aminotransferase
AST	aspartate aminotransferase
bd	twice daily
BP	blood pressure
bpm	beats per minute
BUN	blood urea nitrogen
CBC	complete blood count
CHF	congestive heart failure
CK	creatine kinase
CK-MB	creatine kinase isoenzyme found predominantly in myocardial cells
co-amoxiclav	clavulanate-potentiated amoxicillin
co-codamol	paracetamol and codeine
co-magaldrox	mixture of magnesium hydroxide and aluminium salts
CRP	C-reactive protein
CXR	chest radiograph
DH	drug history
DNA	deoxyribonucleic acid
DVT	deep vein thrombosis
ec	enteric coated
ECG	electrocardiogram
EEG	electroencephalography
ESR	erythrocyte sedimentation rate
FH	family history
GFR	glomerular filtration rate
GGT	gamma-glutamyl transpeptidase
GORD	gastro-oesophageal reflux disease
h	hour
HbA1c	glycosylated haemoglobin
HIV	human immunodeficiency virus
HMG-CoA	3-hydroxyl-3-methyglutaryl coenzyme A

im	intramuscular
INR	international normalised ratio
iv	intravenous
K	potassium
LDL	low-density-lipoprotein cholesterol
LFTs	liver function tests
L	left
LMWH	low-molecular-weight heparin
MCH	mean corpuscular haemoglobin
MCHC	mean corpuscular haemoglobin concentration
MCV	mean corpuscular volume
Na	sodium
nocte	at night
NSAID	non-steroidal anti-inflammatory drug
°	no (absence of)
O/E	on examination
po	via oral route
PC	presenting complaint
PMH	past medical history
prn	as required
qid	four times daily
QT interval in ECG	the time between depolarisation and polarisation of the ventricles
R	right
RBC	red blood cells
SH	social history
SOB	shortness of breath
SSRI	selective serotonin re-uptake inhibitor
FT$_4$	free thyroxine
TCA	tricyclic antidepressant
tds	three times daily
TSH	thyroid stimulating hormone
U&Es	urea and electrolytes
UV	ultraviolet
WBC	white blood cells

Appendix C

Clinical laboratory tests reference limits

Normal ranges for laboratory tests vary significantly depending on the method of testing and the laboratory. The values reported here are for the adult population and are indicative of normal values.

Alanine aminotransferase	8–20 U/l
Alkaline phosphatase	42–128 U/l
Aspartate aminotransferase	5–40 IU/l
Bilirubin, total, blood	5.1–17.0 mmol/l
Blood glucose, fasting	3.6–6.0 mmol/l
Blood glucose, random	<7.8 mmol/l
Blood pressure	120/80 mmHg
BUN	3.6–7.1 mmol/l
Chloride, blood	96–106 mmol/l
Cholesterol	<5.20 mmol/l
Creatine kinase	<175 U/l
Creatinine, blood	50–110 µmol/l
ESR	< 30 mm/hr
Gamma-glutamyl transpeptidase	8–38 U/l
Haemoglobin	7.4–9.9 mmol/l
HbA1c	4–8%
HDL	>0.75 mmol/l
LDL	<3.37 mmol/l
MCV	80–95 mm^3
MCH	27–31 pg
MCHC	32–36 g/dl
pH	7.1
Platelets	150–400 × 10^9/l
Potassium, blood	3.5–5.0 mmol/l
Pulse	60–80 beats/minute
Red blood cell count	4.4–5.8 × 10^{12}/l
Sodium, blood	135–145 mmol/l
Thyroxine T$_4$	4–12 µg/dl
Thyroxine, free	0.8–2.7 ng/dl

Temperature, body	37°C (98.6°F)
Thyroid-stimulating hormone	2–10 mU/l
Triglyceride	0.40–1.52 mmol/l
Urea	3.0–8.0 mmol/l
Uric acid	0.15–0.48 mmol/l
White blood cell count	5–10.0 × 10⁹/l

Appendix D

Performance statistics

Tests 1 to 4 were undertaken by a sample of final-year pharmacy students following a five-year undergraduate course. The percentage of students answering a question incorrectly is indicated for each test. For each test, the median score obtained by the student group is presented.

Test 1 (n = 23)

Median score obtained: 46% (range 37–53%)

Question number	Students answering incorrectly (%)
1	18
2	11
3	49
4	11
5	0
6	0
7	33
8	91
9	38
10	62
11	18
12	20
13	40
14	27
15	4
16	31
17	42
18	22
19	42
20	73

Test 1 (n = 23) (continued)

Question number	Students answering incorrectly (%)
21	22
22	16
23	18
24	61
25	47
26	42
27	7
28	64
29	16
30	7
31	18
32	2
33	9
34	69
35	60
36	17
37	24
38	11
39	11
40	0
41	24
42	24
43	20
44	31
45	29
46	4
47	7
48	2
49	11
50	11
51	24
52	18

Test 1 (n = 23) (continued)

Question number	Students answering incorrectly (%)
53	22
54	4
55	38
56	33
57	58
58	9
59	0
60	7
61	36
62	89
63	84
64	11
65	96
66	64
67	54
68	9
69	57
70	12
71	4
72	8
73	15
74	21
75	83
76	78
77	17
78	4
79	22
80	78

Test 2 (n = 24)

Median score obtained: 58% (range 51–66%)

Question number	Students answering incorrectly (%)
1	0
2	4
3	8
4	8
5	0
6	17
7	0
8	71
9	29
10	29
11	54
12	17
13	75
14	0
15	38
16	42
17	4
18	88
19	17
20	25
21	25
22	8
23	25
24	17
25	50
26	13
27	8
28	17
29	0
30	17

Test 2 (n = 24) (continued)

Question number	Students answering incorrectly (%)
31	71
32	33
33	42
34	8
35	4
36	0
37	38
38	0
39	71
40	13
41	29
42	13
43	8
44	4
45	0
46	0
47	4
48	33
49	29
50	21
51	75
52	21
53	29
54	0
55	25
56	33
57	38
58	79
59	8
60	38
61	4
62	17

Test 2 (n = 24) (continued)

Question number	Students answering incorrectly (%)
63	4
64	50
65	13
66	22
67	87
68	57
69	65
70	39
71	74
72	30
73	77
74	19
75	15
76	13
77	63
78	25
79	13
80	21

Test 3 (n = 53)

Median score obtained: 66% (range 40–86%)

Question number	Students answering incorrectly (%)
1	21
2	8
3	74
4	28
5	45
6	11

Test 3 (n = 53) (continued)

Question number	Students answering incorrectly (%)
7	32
8	40
9	47
10	28
11	28
12	23
13	30
14	30
15	83
16	25
17	40
18	40
19	40
20	6
21	6
22	34
23	60
24	47
25	42
26	28
27	8
28	59
29	25
30	19
31	43
32	36
33	15
34	62
35	13
36	38
37	25
38	28

Test 3 (n = 53) (continued)

Question number	Students answering incorrectly (%)
39	50
40	9
41	49
42	17
43	11
44	13
45	47
46	8
47	62
48	9
49	11
50	72
51	19
52	64
53	34
54	77
55	9
56	21
57	32
58	38
59	75
60	59
61	13
62	26
63	19
64	38
65	23
66	30
67	53
68	21
69	74
70	28

Test 3 (n = 53) (continued)

Question number	Students answering incorrectly (%)
71	8
72	57
73	47
74	28
75	47
76	68
77	30
78	9
79	6
80	51

Test 4 (n = 23)

Median score obtained: 56% (range 46–76%)

Question number	Students answering incorrectly (%)
1	0
2	9
3	0
4	22
5	39
6	74
7	39
8	70
9	13
10	48
11	22
12	26
13	39
14	39

Test 4 (n = 23) (continued)

Question number	Students answering incorrectly (%)
15	52
16	44
17	30
18	78
19	39
20	74
21	9
22	39
23	61
24	22
25	52
26	30
27	30
28	48
29	44
30	52
31	39
32	26
33	83
34	70
35	9
36	35
37	30
38	22
39	57
40	65
41	30
42	57
43	13
44	83
45	35
46	4

Test 4 (n = 23) (continued)

Question number	Students answering incorrectly (%)
47	57
48	70
49	22
50	9
51	44
52	35
53	74
54	65
55	83
56	83
57	96
58	52
59	96
60	22
61	52
62	61
63	13
64	39
65	57
66	78
67	65
68	65
69	18
70	22
71	52
72	44
73	44
74	9
75	70
76	13
77	9
78	26

Test 4 (n = 23) (continued)

Question number	Students answering incorrectly (%)
79	44
80	4

Generic drug names index

Explanation of page references in all four indexes:
First number refers to an answer.
Number in parens refers to the corresponding question.
Where there are two numbers in parens, the first one refers to the preamble to the question.

Conditions index

abdominal discomfort, 101, 103, (133), 160

abdominal pain, (13), 51, 89, 150 (119)

acid regurgitation, 196 (173)

acidosis, metabolic, 34–35 (4)

acne, 36, 143

addiction, opioids, 34 (4)

adenocarcinoma, 146, 194

agitation, 208, 209

agranulocytosis, (66), 145

akathisia, (66)

alcoholism, 42–43 (11–2)

alkalosis, 91

allergic rhinitis, 42, 92, 93 (60), 190, 219–221 (190–1)

allergies, (20), 29, 97–8 (65–6), 103, 151–2 (120–1)

alopecia, 90, 147 (118)

anaemia, 29 (1), 107–108 (76–7), 143, 166 (137), 201 (176), 204–5 (181)

anaphylaxis, 33–4, 91 (59), (124)

angina, 33, 54 (27), 89 (58), 94 (62), 156–7 (127, 128), 162, 164, 194–5, 210–3 (184, 185–6), 213–6 (186–8) *see also* cardiovascular disease; ischaemic heart disease

anorexia, 46, 49, 109, 144–145

anovulatory infertility, 34

anxiety, 89 (58), 112–114 (81–3)

aortic stenosis, 162

aphasia, 31 (2)

appendicitis, 58

arrhythmias, 54, 87 (57), 144 (116), 203, 207–8 (181–2) 212–3 *see also* atrial fibrillation

asthma, 36–7 (5), 92–93 (60), 114, 151–156 (120–7), 201–204 (177, 178), 221 (190, 191)

ataxia, 95 (63)

atherosclerosis, 88 (57), 100–101, 157

atonic colon, 101 (69)

atopic eczema, 111–112 (80–1), 200 (175)

atrial fibrillation, 46 (15, 16), 201–4 (177–8)

bacterial endocarditis, 47–49 (19)

benign prostatic hyperplasia, 207–208

biliary colic, 89 (58), 150

bleeding, 30, 31, 35, 44 (14), 107–8, 114, 158, 201, 212 (185), 216

blurred vision, 42 (11), 91 (59)

bone marrow suppression, 147, 166, 167 (138), 206 (181)

bowel obstruction, 195

bradycardia, 95, 208

bradykinesia, 110 (77, 79)

breast carcinoma, tamoxifen, 104–105 (72)

breathlessness, 30 (1, 2), 93–97 (60–5), 156–157 (127, 128)

bronchoconstriction, anaphylaxis, 91 (59)

bronchospasm, (8), 149, 152 (120–1), 202

bruising, 30

Subject index

Cases index